# Leadership, Branding, and the Business of Dermatology

*Editor*

TERRENCE A. CRONIN JR.



DERMATOLOGIC CLINICS

www.derm.theclinics.com

*Consulting Editor*
BRUCE H. THIERS

October 2026 • Volume 44 • Number 4

**ELSEVIER**

1818 Market Street • Suite 3323 • Philadelphia, Pennsylvania, 19103-2899

http://www.theclinics.com

**DERMATOLOGIC CLINICS Volume 44, Number 4**
**October 2026 ISSN 0733-8635, ISBN-13: 978-0-443-42965-1**

Editor: Stacy Eastman
Developmental Editor: Nitesh Barthwal



**Publishing Office:** *Dermatologic Clinics* (ISSN 0733-8635) is published quarterly by Elsevier Inc., 1818 Market Street, Philadelphia, PA 19103, United States. Periodicals postage paid at New York, NY and additional mailing offices. USA POSTMASTER: Send address changes to *Dermatologic Clinics*, Elsevier Customer Service Department, 3251 Riverport Lane, Maryland Heights, MO 63043, USA. Months of publication are January, April, July, and October. Subscription prices are USD 456.00 per year for US individuals, USD 488.00 per year for Canadian individuals, USD 558.00 per year for international individuals, USD 100.00 per year for US students/residents, USD 100.00 per year for Canadian students/residents, and USD 240 per year for international students/residents. For institutional access pricing please contact Customer Service via the contact information below. International air speed delivery is included in all *Clinics* subscription prices. All prices are subject to change without notice. Orders, claims, and journal inquiries: Please visit our Support Hub page https://service.elsevier.com for assistance.

*Reprints.* For copies of 100 or more, of articles in this publication, please contact the Commercial Reprints Department, Elsevier Inc., 360 Park Avenue South, New York, New York 10010-1710. Tel.: 212-633-3874; Fax: 212-633-3820; Email: reprints@elsevier.com.

The *Dermatologic Clinics* is covered in *MEDLINE/PubMed (Index Medicus)*, *Current Contents/Clinical Medicine, Excerpta Medica, Chemical Abstracts,* and *ISI/BIOMED*.

# Contributors


## CONSULTING EDITOR

**BRUCE H. THIERS, MD**
Professor and Chairman Emeritus, Department of Dermatology and Dermatologic Surgery, Medical University of South Carolina, Charleston, South Carolina

## EDITOR

**TERRENCE A. CRONIN Jr, MD, FAAD**
Associate Voluntary Professor, Frost Department of Dermatology and Cutaneous Surgery, University of Miami, Miami, Florida; Owner, Cronin Skin Cancer Center, Melbourne, Florida

## AUTHORS

**OYETEWA ASEMPA, MD, FAAD**
Director, Skin of Color Clinic, Assistant Professor, Department of Dermatology, Baylor College of Medicine, Houston, Texas

**SYNCLAIR BAKER, MS**
Independent Consultant, Melbourne, Florida

**BROOKE BARTLEY, MD**
Melanoma and Cutaneous Oncology Research Fellow, Department of Dermatology, University of Texas Southwestern Medical Center, Dallas, Texas

**M. HUNTER BOHMAN, DO**
Melanoma and Cutaneous Oncology Research Fellow, Department of Dermatology, University of Texas Southwestern Medical Center, Dallas, Texas

**CHERYL BURGESS, MD, FAAD**
Assistant Clinical Professor, Department of Dermatology, Center for Dermatology and Dermatologic Surgery, Washington, DC

**CLAY J. COCKERELL, MD, MBA, JD**
Founder and President, Cockerell Dermatopathology, Program Director, HES/ Lake Granbury Dermatology Residency, Clinical Professor, Department of Dermatology and Dermatopathology, UT Southwestern Medical Center, Dallas, Texas

**MEGAN CRONIN, MD, FAAD**
Dermatologist, Cronin Skin Cancer Center, Melbourne, Florida

**TERRENCE A. CRONIN Jr, MD, FAAD**
Associate Voluntary Professor, Frost Department of Dermatology and Cutaneous Surgery, University of Miami, Miami, Florida; Owner, Cronin Skin Cancer Center, Melbourne, Florida

**SEEMAL R. DESAI, MD, FAAD**
Founder and Medical Director, Innovative Dermatology, Clinical Associate Professor, Department of Dermatology, University of Texas Southwestern Medical Center, Dallas, Texas

**CHARLES L. DUNN, MD, FAAD, FAAP**
Board Certified Dermatologist, Mohs Micrographic Surgeon, Pediatrician, Assistant Professor, Department of Dermatology, KCU / GME Consortium, Advanced Dermatology and Cosmetic Surgery, Port Orange, Florida

**RONDA FARAH, MD FAAD, CEO**
Alluma Dermatology PLLC, Medina, Minnesota; Department of Dermatology, University of Minnesota, Minneapolis, Minnesota

**KATHY FIELDS, MD**
Adjunct Clinical Professor, Department of Dermatology, Stanford University School of Medicine, Redwood City, California; Private Practice, San Francisco, California

**LORENA OLIVEIRA FONSECA, MD**
Research Fellow, Department of Dermatology, University of Minnesota, Alluma Dermatology, Minneapolis, Minnesota

**MELANIE HALL, BSJ**
Senior Vice President, Growth, Brand and Partnerships, Communication and Marketing, American Academy of Dermatology, Rosemont, Illinois

**BRITANY HARTSHORN, BS**
Osteopathic Medical Student, Burrell College of Health Sciences, School of Osteopathic Medicine, Melbourne, Florida

**GEORGE J. HRUZA, MD, MBA**
Adjunct Professor, Department of Dermatology, St. Louis University, St Louis, Missouri; Representative, Missouri State House; Schweiger Dermatology Group, Chesterfield, Missouri

**ARIANNE SHADI KOUROSH, MD, MPH**
Associate Professor, Department of Dermatology, Harvard Medical School, Associate Professor of Environmental Health, Harvard TH Chan School of Public Health, Beth Israel Deaconess Medical Center, Boston, Massachusetts

**YIWEN HELEN LI, MD, MS**
Resident Physician, Department of Dermatology, Emory University School of Medicine, Atlanta, Georgia

**CHRISTIAN MacDONALD, BS**
Medical Student, Florida State University College of Medicine, Tallahassee, Florida

**ANAR MIKAILOV, MD, FAAD**
Board-Certified Dermatologist, Schweiger Dermatology Group, Brighton, New York

**SARA MOGHADDAM, MD, FAAD**
Board Certified Dermatologist, Mohs Micrographic Surgeon, Delmarva Skin Specialists, Selbyville, Delaware

**SABINE OBAGI, MD**
Preliminary Internal Medicine Resident (PGY-1), Department of Internal Medicine, Harbor-UCLA Medical Center, David Geffen School of Medicine at UCLA, Torrance, California

**KATHERINE PLAMPTON, MD**
Research Fellow, Alluma Dermatology, Minneapolis, Minnesota

**SRDJAN PRODANOVICH, MD, FAAD**
Board-Certified Dermatologist, Department of Dermatology, Advanced Dermatologic and Cosmetic Institute, Naples, Florida

**BRITTANI REMÉ, DO, MS**
Research Fellow, Department of Dermatology, Baylor College of Medicine, Houston, Texas

**DARRELL S. RIGEL, MD, MS**
Adjunct Professor, Department of Dermatology, University of Texas Southwestern Medical Center, Dallas, Texas; Clinical Professor of Dermatology, NYU Grossman School of Medicine, New York, New York; Consultant Dermatologist, Cooper Clinic, Dallas, Texas

**KATIE RODAN, MD**
Independent Contractor, Department of Dermatology, Stanford University School of Medicine, Redwood City, California

**ESTHER WOJCICKI, PhD (hc)**
Educator, Author, and Leadership Mentor, Palo Alto, California

# Contents

# DERMATOLOGIC CLINICS

## FORTHCOMING ISSUES

*January 2027*
**New and Emerging Infectious Diseases**
John Trinidad, *Editor*

*April 2027*
**Advances in Medical Dermatology**
Michelle Tarbox, *Editor*

*July 2027*
**Wounds and Wound Healing, Part I**
Hadar Lev-Tov and Jose Jaller, *Editors*

## RECENT ISSUES

*July 2026*
**Medical Devices in Dermatology**
Neil S. Sadick and Suleima Arruda, *Editors*

*April 2026*
**What's New in Dermatopathology**
Tammie C. Ferringer, *Editor*

*January 2026*
**Climate Change and its Impact on Dermatology**
Misha Rosenbach and Eva Rawlings Parker, *Editors*

# Preface

# Leadership, Branding, and the Business of Dermatology

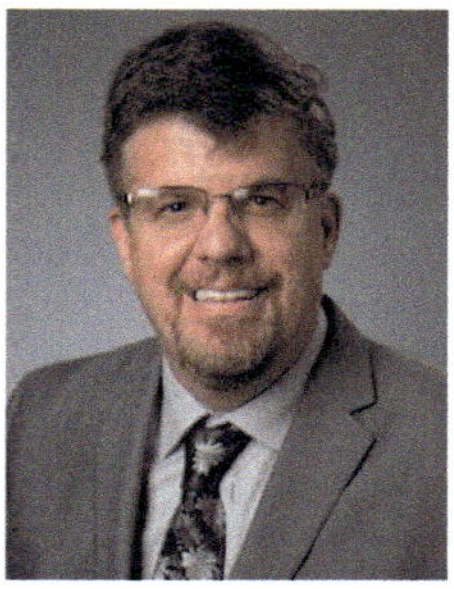

Terrence A. Cronin Jr, MD, FAAD
*Editor*

In the noble pursuit of healing patients with skin diseases, we do far more than treat conditions; we shape confidence, restore health, and transform lives. Yet in today's world, clinical excellence alone is no longer enough. The practice of dermatology has evolved into a multifaceted endeavor where medical mastery must be matched by visionary leadership, intentional branding, and sharp business acumen. This issue of *Dermatologic Clinics* exists at that powerful intersection.

Leadership in dermatology is not about titles or authority; it is about courage. The courage to build cultures of excellence, to mentor the next generation, to innovate treatment protocols, and to champion standards that elevate the entire profession. Great leaders in our field don't just run practices; they inspire movements. They turn clinics into communities and patients into loyal advocates.

Branding, meanwhile, has become a vital form of professional integrity. In an era of social media, aesthetic marketplaces, and informed consumers, your brand is your promise. It is an authentic expression of your expertise, values, and unique approach to care. A strong brand attracts the right patients, builds loyal trust, and differentiates you in a crowded field not through hype, but through clarity, consistency, and dedication.

The business of dermatology is ultimately about sustainability and impact. When practices thrive financially, they can invest in cutting-edge technology, attract top talent, expand access to care, and fund research that pushes our field forward. Profit is not the enemy of purpose; when stewarded wisely, it becomes the fuel for greater purpose.

This issue is designed to be your strategic companion and source of inspiration. Within these pages, you will find actionable insights, real-world examples, leadership frameworks, branding strategies, and business principles specifically tailored to the unique world of dermatology thanks to the many superstar dermatologists who contributed to this incredible issue. Whether you are a solo practitioner building your dream clinic, a medical director overseeing a multilocation practice, or an industry leader shaping the

Dermatol Clin 44 (2026) xi–xii
https://doi.org/10.1016/j.det.2026.07.001

future of dermatologic medicine and surgery, this resource is for you.

The future belongs to those who refuse to choose between being exceptional clinicians and exceptional business leaders. You did not enter this field to merely survive. You entered it to lead, to create, to make a lasting mark. Let this journal be the catalyst that helps you do exactly that.

Welcome to a new era of dermatology where leadership, branding, and business excellence don't just support your patient care expertise but amplify it to your highest potential. Now, turn the page and begin reading. The profession is awaiting your turn to lead.

Stay passionate about Dermatology!

## DISCLOSURES

The author has no conflicts of interest or disclosures.

Terrence A. Cronin Jr, MD, FAAD
Frost Department of Dermatology and Cutaneous Surgery
University of Miami, Miami, FL, USA

Cronin Skin Cancer Center
1399 South Harbor City Boulevard
Melbourne, FL 32901, USA

*E-mail address:*
TCronin2@aol.com

# Company, Product Development and Branding (Proactiv Solution, Rodan + Fields)

Kathy Fields, MD[a,b,*], Katie Rodan, MD[c], Synclair Baker, MS[d]

**KEYWORDS**

• Dermatology • Entrepreneurship • Skincare branding • Proactiv solution • Rodan + fields
• Product development

**KEY POINTS**

- Proactiv Solution and Rodan + Fields Skincare transformed consumer skincare through innovative regimen-based systems with clinically meaningful outcomes.
- Dermatology-driven entrepreneurship requires a strong unwavering mission, market insight, and strategic timing.
- Brand success depends on formulation excellence, marketing innovation, and authentic consumer connection.

> *"The most important real estate you will ever own is your face. It is your calling card to the world; it reflects your confidence. As dermatologists, it is our responsibility to heal and protect this most valuable asset."*
>
> *Dr Kathy Fields and Dr Katie Rodan*

## INTRODUCTION

Against all odds, how could 2 dermatologists with humble beginnings and no business experience defy industry standards by prioritizing performance over profits, loyalty over ego, and integrity above all to create 2 separate billion-dollar brands?

The field of dermatology has witnessed a remarkable evolution in product development and branding, specifically in the consumer skincare market. The groundbreaking stories of Proactiv Solution and Rodan + Fields serve as compelling case studies in dermatologic entrepreneurship. Founded by Dr Katie Rodan and Dr Kathy Fields, both companies revolutionized skincare by tackling issues from acne to aging with innovative formulas and strategic marketing. Their systems represented a paradigm shift in over-the-counter skin care. They did not spot treat problems; instead, they employed a multimedication approach within a simple full-face skincare regimen. By treating and preventing various skin concerns, they achieved transformative results, to the delight and devotion of their customers.[1,2]

## DISCUSSION

### *Building the Brands*

#### *Proactiv solution (1995–2016)*

The story begins in 1984 at Stanford University, where Drs Katie Rodan and Kathy Fields met during their dermatology residency. Upon completing

[a] Department of Dermatology, Stanford University School of Medicine, Redwood City, CA, USA; [b] Private Practice, San Francisco, CA, USA; [c] Department of Dermatology, Stanford University School of Medicine, Redwood City, CA, USA; [d] Independent Consultant, Melbourne, FL, USA
* Corresponding author. 2100 Webster Street, Suite 505, San Francisco, CA 94123.
*E-mail address:* kats1@me.com

Dermatol Clin 44 (2026) 541–547
https://doi.org/10.1016/j.det.2026.06.006

| Abbreviation | |
|---|---|
| AI | artificial intelligence |

their residency, the 2 became practicing dermatologists in the Bay Area in 1987 and remained close friends.

By 1989, Rodan and Fields identified a problem with access to medical care, as health maintenance organizations frequently denied coverage for medications and dermatologic care. At the time, there was a lack of effective over-the-counter acne treatments, and prescription medicines were too harsh for patients to stay on for long-term compliance. Insurance companies believed the acne arena was unimportant as the market size was small and teenagers were noncompliant. Insurance companies stopped access to care, specifically for people over the age of 21 years, with the misguided dogma that people grew out of the disease. Despite insurance companies' beliefs, Drs Rodan and Fields knew that acne was a significant concern, far greater than the 3% reported in the literature for adult women.[3] They also knew it was more than a vanity concern, as it can impair people emotionally and physically, leaving scars for life.[2,4]

With the problem identified, the women took the advice of Dr Eugene Farber, former Chairman of Dermatology at Stanford, to heart: "Get a hobby, or you will be doomed to treating acne and warts." In 1990, the 2 women were compelled to take action and signed a 5 sentence contract, declaring themselves "50/50 partners" in developing a new acne solution. This solution was designed to create elegant, preventive acne formulas that are PROactive, not REactive. The pair self-funded the endeavor, keeping spending minimal and tightly controlled. Rodan and Fields naively set out to make that formula in Dr Rodan's kitchen!

In 1993, after years of failed formulas, the pair found a chemist in New York who could bring their vision to life with excellence. Together, they created and clinically tested a novel low-strength, 3 medicine regimen-based system for daily use on the whole face.[1] The regimen protected the skin's barrier, a first, and was a pleasure to use with a clean nonsensitizing fragrance. Upon completing the clinical trial for their product, the dermatologists pitched Proactiv Solution to the beauty brand Neutrogena. Neutrogena was the "Dermatologist Recommended" brand at the time. Negotiations lasted a year but collapsed when Johnson & Johnson bought Neutrogena.

In 1995, Rodan and Fields licensed their product to Guthy-Renker, the industry leader in the new direct marketing business and an expert in the emerging world of television infomercials. This move was a risky, forward-thinking marketing opportunity that other "high-integrity" businesses had looked down on. However, it was this strategic partnership with Guthy-Renker, which managed the production, distribution, and marketing of Proactiv Solution, that truly brought the product to the consumer. Celebrity endorsements were channel stoppers, but the before-and-afters plus authentic testimonials compelled consumers to buy. The company offered a full money back guarantee if it failed to work. The doctors' formulas and this new marketing format demonstrated the power of collaboration in business.

Proactiv Solution quickly became a market leader and, over the following decade, evolved into a billion-dollar brand. By addressing a substantial unmet need with an effective, accessible regimen, the product achieved widespread consumer adoption. Proactiv Solution disrupted the traditional acne treatment landscape, which had been largely dominated by prescription therapies and office-based care, by demonstrating that a regimen-based over-the-counter approach could effectively manage acne for many consumers.[1,5] Its success coincided with a broader shift toward consumer-directed acne care and highlighted the growing role of over-the-counter therapies in dermatologic treatment.[2,4]

## *Rodan + Fields (2003–2007, 2008–2022)*

Early on, with the success of their multimedication approach, the doctors decided to pursue a new venture that targeted concerns such as sun damage, rosacea, and sensitivity, particularly among adult women. In 2003, they launched a second concurrent company, Rodan + Fields. Ironically, Guthy-Renker was not interested in this new opportunity. Despite this, Rodan + Fields was quickly acquired by Estée Lauder in 2003. Estée Lauder utilized traditional retail methods to sell the Rodan + Fields line in department stores. However, the placement failed to reflect the brand's potential amid the decline in department store foot traffic and internal neglect within the Estée Lauder conglomerate. Thus, sales were slow to materialize. The company's iron-fisted control over its products and complicated overhead sharing scheme left the founders with no chance for success. So the doctors had the courage and commitment to buy back their company and operate independently in 2007. This was a testament to their belief in the products and the need to reach customers. It was also a testament to their entrepreneurial spirit and resilience.

In 2008, the Rodan + Fields brand re-emerged under the full ownership of Drs Rodan and Fields. This iteration represented a central entrepreneurial pivot, utilizing a radically different business model–network marketing. The timing coincided with the Great Recession, and their vision was simple yet powerful: empower the women who loved, trusted, and used the products to participate directly in their distribution and success.

Through this model, women became independent consultants, their own bosses, and earned their own money to achieve financial security. People at any level of education could achieve unlimited wealth if they worked hard. By 2011, the convergence of smartphones, Facebook, and a growing appetite for flexible income opportunities helped propel Rodan + Fields into unicorn status by 2018. Unlike traditional retail brands, their consultants became brand ambassadors, today's influencers, blending e-commerce with authenticity.[6,7]

At one point, 300,000 consultants were on board. The approach expanded the brand's reach while fostering peer-driven engagement and loyalty. Beyond commercial success, Drs Rodan and Fields regard the communities formed by the independent consultants—and their sustained partnership with one another—as among the most meaningful and enduring outcomes of the company's legacy. The doctors had attracted people who wanted to help others live well in their skin and in their personal lives. Indeed, the consultants supported each other through cancer, divorce, and millions of difficulties.

The 2 companies completely upended traditional retail. Rodan and Fields skin care companies were not just a product but a promise of healthy skin. Trust was established through peer education, experiential validation, and visible outcomes, all of which are known drivers of health care brand credibility.[8,9]

## How to Build Your Company

### Doctors as the brand

Every successful product solves a problem. The first step to building your brand is to articulate the problem your product will address. The problem you are trying to solve has to be so compelling that you are willing to devote your life to it. If you are solely motivated by money, you will fail. Entrepreneurship is a long road with many inevitable surprises, setbacks, and no guarantees. Worse still, there are factors beyond your control on both the local and global stage that disrupt all companies and can cause you to lose momentum. Thus, a clear and compelling "Why" can become the anchor that sustains entrepreneurs through these challenging times.

Doctors today want to be the Brand. Many are selling their virtual lives on social media to be famous and hope for monetary gains. They are white-labeling products and jumping into the red ocean of TikTok. This is not a sustainable venture. A few may rise above the noise to garner a following, yet, without a life-enhancing proposition and strong follow-through, that customer will move on to the next shiny thing. There will always be the next best thing.

Key questions to answer:

- What specific issue does your product address?
- Why is this problem significant?
- How large is the problem in terms of size and dollar share?
- Who is your target audience?
- How does your product offer a better or novel solution than existing treatments?
- Is your idea a "me too" product?
- Are you confident that the need is so vital that you will remain committed to the project?
- Can you protect your idea from knock-offs?

## Forming the Right Partnership

At the heart of Drs Rodan and Fields' success in their companies was a deeply aligned partnership built on trust, shared values, and complementary strengths. Long before their first product was developed, they had already laid the groundwork for one of dermatologic history's most powerful and influential entrepreneurial alliances. Their strong partnership turned a vision into velocity, with trust fueling progress and shared purpose driving results.

Rodan and Fields aligned themselves from the start, not just in their medical discipline but also in their purpose. They did not set out to build a skincare empire for the sake of wealth. Their "why" was rooted in patients' needs, filling a gap where traditional dermatology fell short. They filled this gap by democratizing medical care and delivering on-demand results without a prescription. This shared purpose served as the compass that guided every major decision. From rejecting offers that did not align with their values, to buying back Rodan + Fields from Estée Lauder when it no longer fulfilled their vision. They had a mantra. "Your reputation is your most powerful ingredient," so "Do The Right Thing."

Despite all their success, they were not without their conflicts, as they are 2 strong-willed, laser-focused women. This clarity of purpose made it easier to overcome those conflicts and stay the course. Outside stressors often tried to disrupt the doctors' relationship. Thus, the doctors sought professional counseling to keep their relationship on track. They realized their relationship was a cornerstone of their brand's resilience and clarity of vision. Doctors Rodan and Fields further acknowledged that if divided, they would fall, and they could not let that happen.

Key questions to answer:

- Do you and your partner(s) share a clear, common purpose?
- What strengths does each partner bring—and where are the gaps?
- How will you handle conflict, growth, and decision-making?
- Are you committed to preserving the partnership amid evolving challenges?

## *Identify the Market Size and Opportunity*

Do your homework before you create a product! Thorough market research is essential to building a successful skincare brand. It is not enough to have a great product—you must also determine whether there is a large enough demand to support business growth. Examining the demand involves assessing market size, consumer behavior, industry trends, and the competitive landscape. Artificial intelligence (AI) has been a game-changer in quickly finding these answers and with some degree of certainty. AI is the future of creating a skincare line with the click of a button. It looks brilliant on a computer, except it cannot execute the many parts of a well-rounded company.

The global skincare industry, specifically, is a multibillion-dollar market that continues to expand. The skincare industry is fueled by increasing consumer awareness, advancements in dermatologic research, and a growing demand for personalized beauty solutions. This vast industry is diverse and segmented and covers multiple skin concerns. However, it is also a highly competitive, noisy arena, making it difficult to rise above the rest.

The dermatologists had a unique advantage. With their expertise in dermatology, pathophysiology, skincare formulations, and understanding of the consumer psyche, doctors Rodan and Fields deeply understood what was needed to create an impactful and sustainable product. Their firsthand experience with patients allowed them to pinpoint the most pressing concerns.

Key questions to answer:

- How large is the market for your product?
- Is it a fad or a trend? For example, salmon sperm and snail slime are the ingredients de jour. They are unlikely to last 40 years like retinol has.
- Is this market growing? Will the problem addressed be prevalent in the years to come?
- What market segment does your brand target (eg, acne, antiaging, sensitive skin, teens, women, men, and children)? The segment of preteens using luxury skincare is small and transient. Would you be willing to gamble in that market?
- Are you splitting or lumping groups? Splitters will focus on hair loss with pseudo-folliculitis barbae, while lumpers will strive to help everyone who shaves.
- Do you have a cure or a preventive strategy that will keep people using the product continuously?
- Are you willing to adapt as trends, platforms, and consumer preferences evolve?
- What is your unique value proposition? What is your core promise of unique value? Is it your ingredient, philosophy, or results that would make someone choose you over all the rest?
- TikTok is last year's marketing platform—are you willing to reach for the new and emerging platforms? Can you beat AI?

## *Define Ownership and Investment Structure*

Defining ownership and investment structure is among the most consequential strategic decisions in building a dermatology-driven company. This choice influences not only financial outcomes but also governance, control, scalability, and the founder's ability to remain aligned with the original mission. Decisions made early—often before a product reaches the market—can shape a company's trajectory for decades and are difficult, if not impossible, to reverse.

Entrepreneurs must decide whether to self-fund, seek external investment, or pursue strategic partnerships.[10] Self-funding offers maximum control but may limit early growth, while external capital can accelerate expansion at the cost of equity dilution and shared decision-making. The right investors can add significant value by professionalizing operations and providing strategic expertise; however, for physician-founders, this trade-off is especially consequential, as outside pressures may conflict with medical integrity, patient-centered values, and long-term brand trust. A critical self-assessment is recognizing that founders often "do not know what they do not know," making mentorship not optional but essential throughout the entrepreneurial journey.

Drs Rodan and Fields managed risk with exceptional discipline, retaining control over major decisions and avoiding unnecessary expenditures. In the early stages, they relied on their dermatology practices as a financial safety net while developing their products—an approach that underscores the importance of realistically assessing one's financial cushion. Not all entrepreneurs can afford to abandon clinical practice prematurely. While self-funding requires personal financial commitment and careful risk management, the success of Proactiv Solution and Rodan + Fields demonstrates that when ownership decisions are aligned with mission, fiscal discipline, and mentorship, founders can build enduring brands with both clinical credibility and substantial commercial impact.

Key questions to answer:

- Who owns the company?
- Who can advise you on creating a corporate structure relevant to your vision? You will need an attorney and an accountant to set up your business as an LLC, S Corp, C Corp, or another entity. It is vital to start correctly. The investors will come in, and this will create a capitalization table. You must get this set up professionally because your company will evolve. This is not the time to use AI for a contract!
- Can you own your intellectual property? It is vital to have protected and patented IP.
- Are you prepared to assume the financial risk of building your business?
- Can you fund product development, marketing, and distribution on your own?
- Do you have a safety net or alternative income source while building your brand?

## *Identify the Competition*

Achieving true innovation requires the courage to be a disruptor—challenging traditional methods, redefining industry standards, and taking calculated risks. This type of breakthrough does not happen by chance; it requires guidance and expertise from consultants with in-depth knowledge of the field.

In marketing, there are 2 oceans—red and blue. The red ocean is a shark-infested bloodbath of competition, where companies capitalize on the leftovers of big brands by targeting established competitors in a well-known market. An example is small knock-off brands of market leaders, such as Acne Free, which claimed to be "better than Proactiv." Yet, despite this claim, it ultimately led to an increase in Proactiv Solution sales. On the other hand, the blue ocean strategy stimulates businesses to venture into uncharted territory, establishing new markets through creative thinking and originality. The goal in the blue ocean is to be first and fast before others catch on, while also being willing to take the risk. Understanding these strategies can help you position your brand effectively.

The courageous disruptors boldly dove into the blue ocean strategy, venturing into untapped spaces with a unique product platform and distribution models. They recognized their success depended on differentiation rather than direct competition from other skincare brands. Proactiv Solution would not have been discovered if it were under the Neutrogena name, sitting on a low shelf in the drugstore. Likewise, Rodan + Fields did not sit in the shadows of legacy brands at the department store; it became a platform for empowerment, creating thousands of microentrepreneurs and delivering transformative skin results.

Key questions to answer:

- Who are your direct competitors? What are their strengths and weaknesses?
- How will your brand position itself against the competition?
- How will you reach your customers and better serve them than the competition?
- How will you protect your innovation (eg, patents, trademarks, exclusive technology, or proprietary formulas)?

## *Selling Your Product*

Sales are not just about getting a product in someone's hands—they are about creating trust, delivering results, and making the customer feel seen. Drs Rodan and Fields reimagined how skin care could be delivered by choosing marketing channels that aligned with both the product's message and the customer's experience.[6,8]

Unlike most skincare brands, which relied on department stores or pharmacies, Proactiv's subscription-based reorder model, promoted through infomercials, ensured continuous availability and customer retention. Proactiv Solution infomercials served as 30 minute educational programs that explained the underlying causes of acne and emphasized comprehensive, whole-face treatment. Striking before-and-after images, paired with credible consumer testimonials and reinforced by a no-risk, money-back guarantee, created a compelling message. Consumers could order the product directly from the infomercial or later through the brand's Web site and toll-free numbers, making the purchasing accessible and seamless. As antiquated as this seems today, this was a breakthrough achievement in the 1990s.

Proactiv Solution masterfully utilized celebrity testimonials from stars like Judith Light, Vanessa Williams, Jessica Simpson, Katy Perry, and Adam Levine, positioning the brand as a trusted, aspirational solution. These endorsements added credibility and made consumers feel that if Proactiv Solution worked for celebrities, it could work for them as well.

Leveraging various platforms was another key to selling their products. When Rodan + Fields later pivoted to a direct sales model, they recognized the power of social selling and the value of personal recommendations. This method enabled everyday consumers to become brand advocates, creating a grassroots marketing movement built on trust and word of mouth. By offering a direct sales model, they minimized overhead costs while maximizing revenue potential through a commission-based structure. This incentivized consultants to sell and ensured the brand's steady expansion. This was a new paradigm in the 2010s.

Ultimately, Rodan + Fields' success resulted from combining dermatologic expertise with innovative marketing and sales strategies. Their ability to connect with consumers on a personal level, utilize various promotional channels, and consistently deliver results solidified their position as leaders in the skincare industry.

Key questions to answer:

- Who is your target audience, and how do they shop?
- What distribution channel best aligns with your brand (retail, subscription, and social selling)?
- How will you build trust before asking for a purchase?
- What pricing strategy reflects both your value and your customer's expectations?

## SUMMARY

The remarkable journeys of Proactiv Solution and Rodan + Fields demonstrate that with a powerful "why," a deep understanding of patient needs, and relentless perseverance, dermatologists can transcend the clinic to transform the consumer skincare industry. Dr Katie Rodan and Dr Kathy Fields did not just create products—they built movements by aligning medical credibility with marketing innovation, personal storytelling, and a clear mission to make dermatologic care more accessible.

Their ability to anticipate market shifts, from TV infomercials to social selling, reflects a critical truth in entrepreneurship: success belongs to those who are not only rooted in expertise but also agile and courageous in execution. Whether launching a regimen-based acne solution from a kitchen or empowering thousands of microentrepreneurs through network marketing, Rodan + Fields redefines what it means to be both a physician and a founder, and has had a direct impact on millions of lives.

For aspiring dermatology entrepreneurs, their legacy offers a proven, actionable blueprint: identify a real, persistent problem; develop a safe, effective solution; adapt to changing technologies and consumer behaviors; and protect the integrity of your mission through every pivot. In an industry where platforms and trends shift overnight, the enduring value lies in staying purpose-driven, data-informed, and bold enough to lead the conversation, long before the rest of the world catches on.

## CLINICS CARE POINTS

- Prioritize adherence: Simplicity, tolerability, and patient education are critical determinants of long-term treatment. Success is predicated on compliance.
- Build trust through evidence and transparency: Clinical credibility and clear communication drive patient satisfaction and product success.
- Avoid overreliance on trends: Short-lived ingredients or platforms may not sustain long-term therapeutic or commercial success.
- Value real transformative results over vague claims.
- As a physician entrepreneur, staying true to your training will serve you well in your creation of effective treatments.

## FUNDING

The funders are Kathy Fields and Katie Rodan.

## DISCLOSURE

The authors have nothing to disclose.

## REFERENCES

1. Rodan K, Fields K, Falla TJ. Efficacy of a twice-daily, 3-step, over-the-counter skincare regimen for the treatment of acne vulgaris. Clin Cosmet Invest Dermatol 2017;10:3–9.
2. Decker A, Graber EM. Over-the-counter acne treatments: a review. J Clin Aesthet Dermatol 2023; 16(6):28–37.

3. Collier CN, Harper JC, Cantrell WC, et al. The prevalence of acne in adults 20 years and older. J Am Acad Dermatol 2008;58(1):56–9.

4. Tobiasz A, Nowicka D, Szepietowski JC. Acne Vulgaris—Novel treatment options and factors affecting therapy adherence. J Clin Med 2022;11(24):7535.

5. Mavranezouli I, Daly CH, Welton NJ, et al. A systematic review and network meta-analysis of treatments for acne vulgaris. Br J Dermatol 2022; 187(5):639–49.

6. Ranjith P, Nisansala S, Jayasingha N, et al. Does social media information credibility influence social commerce purchase intention of skincare products? Evidence from Facebook. PLoS One 2025;20(10): e0334126.

7. Szeto MD, Mamo A, Afrin A, et al. Social media in dermatology. Curr Dermatol Rep 2021;10(4): 97–104.

8. Purcarea VL. The impact of marketing strategies in healthcare systems. J Med Life 2019;12(2):93–6.

9. Moorman C, van Heerde HJ, Moreau CP, et al. Marketing in the health care sector: disrupted exchanges and new research directions. J Market 2024;88(1):1–14.

10. Wasserman JD, Chen JT. Physician entrepreneurship in dermatology. Dermatol Clin 2019;37(3): 327–34.

# The Anatomy of Unique Product Development

Anar Mikailov, MD*

**KEYWORDS**

• Entrepreneurship in dermatology • Skincare products • Product development
• Formulation development • Bootstrapping • Business development

**KEY POINTS**

- Identifying a problem is the first step to unique product (solution) development.
- Customers prioritize clinician-backed brands.
- Dermatology physicians have a unique advantage to identify problems as well as to become leaders of skincare brands.

## INTRODUCTION

The skincare industry is undergoing a significant transformation, with the global market projected to reach approximately US$235 billion by 2031. Within this massive landscape, dermatology-led and doctor-developed brands are experiencing faster growth than the broader market, driven by a consumer base that increasingly prioritizes clinical efficacy over traditional marketing.[1]

The time to start a brand in the skincare industry, is now. However, this journey is by no means a "side-hustle"; rather an additional full-time commitment. While the necessary knowledge and expertise are entirely attainable for any accomplished clinician, the transition from physician to entrepreneur can still feel daunting. The goal of this article is to demystify the process and empower more dermatologists to embrace entrepreneurship.

My development journey involve two brands: Skintensive (I founded in 2015) and Boston Skin Science (I cofounded in 2018). From personal experience as well as research and conversations with other founders, successful brands by and large follow five key steps (more detail follows in the "Discussion" section):

1. Identifying a critical gap in the market
2. Identifying the exact customer
3. Conceptualizing and meticulously developing the solution
4. Building a cohesive brand
5. Determine the product-market fit

While the broad skincare market is highly competitive, featuring established players ranging from CeraVe to Drunk Elephant to La Mer, small "niche" brands can find success by focusing on specific, underserved dermatologic gaps. When a new brand successfully addresses a unique clinical challenge—or offers a radically better solution to an everyday problem—that "small" niche can quickly translate into massive market growth.

### *The Global Skincare Market Context*

The modern skincare market is no longer just about esthetics; it is viewed by consumers as a vital component of wellness or "holistic health." Based on recent market research, the overall skincare industry is growing at 6% to 7% per year, fueled by rising disposable incomes and a shift toward preventive routines.[1] Women remain the primary consumers, while men are the fastest growing segment due to increased awareness of sun protection and more interest in antiaging. Of all sales, about 4 out of 10 purchases are made through traditional pharmacies and drugstores,

Brighton, NY, USA
* 21 Framark Dr #552, Victor, NY 14564.
*E-mail address:* anar@skintensive.com

Dermatol Clin 44 (2026) 549–554
https://doi.org/10.1016/j.det.2026.05.001

| Abbreviation | |
|---|---|
| SKU | Stock Keeping Unit |

whereas online channels are the fastest-growing distribution method.[2]

Facial care remains the largest segment (40%), but specialized areas like hair and scalp health (38%) are seeing a surge in dermatologist-recommended solutions for concerns like hair thinning and dry scalp.[3]

Dermatologist-led brands, often categorized under "dermocosmetics," are the fastest-growing sector of the industry with an annual growth rate of 9% to 10% with an estimated market size of US$140 billion by 2031.[4] Dermatologist-led brands occupy a unique "trust-based" niche that bridges the gap between mass-market retail and prescription drugs. In 2026, consumers are increasingly developing an in-depth knowledge of skin care through reputable dermatology social media education. These customers are "skin-literate" and often seek out specific percentages of active ingredients (eg, retinoids) and split-face clinical studies rather than vague promises. Shoppers favor medical-grade brands that prioritize transparency and verifiable outcomes that are reviewed and published.

Important to note—strong adoption of new (and legacy) brands often begins in the dermatology office, where professional guidance lends a level of authority that mass-market brands not found in the office rarely match. This "physician-endorsed" model ensures that the products are "trusted" by the dermatologist.[4]

## DISCUSSION

Every successful brand is built upon the foundation of a successful product. In turn, a successful product must solve a problem—whether it is a pain point the consumer actively recognizes or one they have not yet realized they have. Airbnb, for example, was initially dismissed as a radical idea because it addressed an unrecognized need: the desire to stay in a local's home rather than a traditional hotel. Conversely, the Mighty Patch is a prime example of a product that addressed a highly recognizable problem—acne breakouts—by offering a highly novel solution: hydrocolloid technology as spot treatment.

Drawing from my experience building 2 skincare companies, I have distilled the complex process of brand development into 5 critical steps. While this framework may not cover every conceivable scenario, executing these core elements is essential for any brand to succeed in today's market.

### *Five Steps to Brand Development*

#### *Step 1: define the problem*

> *All truths are easy to understand once they are discovered; the point is to discover them.*
> *—Galileo Galilei*

A standout product is anchored by a clear purpose and a specific problem to solve. While some formulations attempt to do it all—like "Egyptian Magic," which boasts 17 different uses—the most successful products laser-focus on 1 or 2 core issues. Unique product opportunities can be found by addressing much less common problems in large populations, highly recognizable problems within specific niche communities or findings a sweet-spot that combines both. Consider, for example, recurrent fungal infections among wrestlers, disrupted skin barriers and severe dryness in competitive swimmers, or moisture-induced folliculitis in frequent hot yoga practitioners.

*KP Away (Boston Skin Science):* Launched in 2015, this brand was built entirely around treating keratosis pilaris. At the time, the market was saturated with products focused strictly on exfoliation—a trend that largely continues today. However, based on an evaluation of medical literature and direct observations from clinical practice, it became clear that an alternative, non-exfoliative approach was necessary. By pivoting to an emollient over exfoliation, KP Away represented a rather major paradigm shift. This brand serves as a good example of addressing a specific problem (albeit moderately common) within a well-defined, small-to-medium-sized demographic (primarily children and teenagers).

*Skintensive:* Launched in 2018, this brand was developed to specifically address actinic purpura and adjacent dermatologic concerns in individuals aged 65 years and older. While this issue is widely recognized by both dermatologists and patients, existing market solutions were minimal and largely ineffective. Furthermore, at the time of the brand's launch, the "Maturing Skin" category did not formally exist; the industry's largest players were almost exclusively dedicated to "Anti-Aging" lines. Skintensive disrupted this space by approaching the Boomer generation with formulations tailored to their actual physiologic needs—like fortifying thin, fragile skin—rather than selling the illusion of reversed aging. By doing so, the product line established clinical authority in treating bruising and helped pioneer the "Maturing Skin" category. Ultimately, Skintensive serves as a good example of targeting a specific clinical gap within a well-defined, expanding demographic.

*Hero Cosmetics:* Now a massive brand that solved one highly visible problem: the acne breakout. The original Mighty Patch offered a hydrocolloid bandage as an alternative to "popping" pimples. This hyperfocus on "spot-treatment" allowed Hero to dominate the acne-care category.

*SEEN Hair Care:* Founded by Dr Iris Rubin, this brand addressed "skinification of hair" by identifying that many haircare products cause breakouts. By creating noncomedogenic haircare, she filled a niche that traditional beauty brands overlooked.

*Black Girl Sunscreen:* This brand solved the historical problem of traditional sunscreens leaving a visible, chalky white cast on darker skin tones. Founder Shontay Lundy formulated a moisturizing sunscreen that absorbs completely clear on melanin-rich skin. By explicitly identifying an overlooked demographic and solving their specific cosmetic pain point, the brand successfully broke into a highly saturated sun-care market.

### Step 2: define the customer

*A friend to all is a friend to none.*

—*Aristotle*

Attempting to appeal to everyone inevitably leads to appealing to no one. In the early stages of product (not brand) development, specificity is critical. Once your hero Stock Keeping Unit (SKU) captures the attention and trust of a highly targeted demographic, you can introduce adjacent products that address complementary problems. By that point, you will have built an activated, loyal audience eager to purchase your next solution.

*Skintensive:* Rather than broadly targeting "anyone with a bruise," we intentionally narrowed our focus to individuals aged 65 years and older who suffer from frequent bruising of the hands and forearms, clinically defined as actinic purpura. This precision paid off: our first 100 customers fit this exact profile, and today, this core demographic continues to account for over half of our annual sales. By capturing this activated audience early on, we were able to successfully introduce adjacent solutions—such as our Crepe Cream—and we continue to actively innovate within this category.

*Stryke Club:* Instead of "anyone with acne," the target is specifically teenage boys. Dr Sheilagh Maguiness targeted teenage boys—a demographic traditionally ignored by the multistep skincare industry—with simple, effective products for "locker room" hygiene and acne.

*Bubble:* Bubble specifically targets the "first-time" skincare user—predominantly young teens. By focusing on this specific group, they capture a customer base just beginning their skincare journey.

*MÊME:* A French dermo-cosmetic brand acquired by Pierre Fabre that specifically targets patients experiencing skin side effects from cancer treatments.

### Step 3: meticulous product development

*Well done is better than well said.*

—*Benjamin Franklin*

Reliability will always deliver much more than empty rhetoric. Development requires strong partnerships with contract manufacturers and a focus on proprietary formulations that deliver on a promise. Successful "doctor-led" brands are growing much faster than traditional brands because consumers expect authenticity. The product formulation and development stage may be one of the longest, but one of the most important. Product efficacy as well as rheology will be quickly appreciated or rejected by customers. A beautiful facade will crumble if the product does not perform. Respect is ultimately earned through consistency and results. Make clear, factual promises about what your product will do, and then ensure the formulation exceeds those expectations.

Brands like Paula's Choice and The Ordinary have paved the way in ingredient transparency and the customer today has a much great ingredient understanding than in the past.

*Skintensive and KP Away:* As a founder, I evaluated and partnered with multiple manufacturing facilities across the United States, requesting small-batch samples to test their capabilities while building relationships with their in-house chemistry teams. Once we identified the ideal partner, we spent over a year collaborating to engineer the perfect initial version of our hero products. The subsequent 12 months were dedicated exclusively to customer evaluation, rigorous testing, and rapid iteration. When selecting a laboratory, a critical requirement is their ability to adjust formulas swiftly. Facilities with experienced, in-house chemists have the agility to move quickly; conversely, those that outsource this expertise will inevitably cause costly delays.

*Doctor Rogers:* Founded by Dr Heather Rogers, the brand is built on a "less is more" development philosophy, utilizing biodegradable and plant-based ingredients. They meticulously avoid common allergens and irritants found in many healing balms, focusing on purity and sustainability. Every ingredient is chosen specifically for its safety profile in postprocedure recovery. Their hero SKU has only 3 ingredients.

*SkinCeuticals:* Known for their "Duke University Antioxidant Patent," this brand's development is built on precise pH levels and concentration ratios.

Their Vitamin C serums are considered the gold standard because of the meticulous stability required to keep the active ingredients effective. This commitment to clinical parameters ensures professional-grade results.

*Biossance:* This brand sets a benchmark in product development by leveraging synthetic biology to create highly stable, sustainable ingredients. The brand engineered a 100% plant-derived squalane from sugarcane. This meticulous scientific approach allowed them to replace historically unethically sourced ingredients with bioidentical, highly efficacious alternatives, demonstrating how advanced laboratory innovation drives both performance and sustainability.

### Step 4: build the brand

To borrow a phrase from a famous agency, "a product sits on a shelf and does a job; a brand lives in the consumer's mind and commands loyalty."[5]

A strong brand evokes a powerful emotion that ultimately drives purchasing behavior. While this journey began with unique formulations, a product alone is neither a business nor a brand. Rather, the brand is the deep emotional connection our customers have developed with our company and our products. The process of building this brand can be broken down into 4 key components. Ultimately, every business must compile these critical elements into a definitive "Brand Bible," which consists of

- The psychological identity
- Verbal identity
- Visual identity
- Packaging system

**Psychological identity** Is the brand clinical, authoritative, data-driven (eg, SkinCeuticals)?

Is the brand more gentle, nurturing, safe (eg, CeraVe and Aveeno)?

Is it loud and disruptive (eg, DrunkElephant and Topicals)?

Define what the brand does not stand for, or stands against, as well as, what it stands for.

What is the company manifesto, core beliefs, and the promise to the customer?

**Verbal identity** The voice of the brand represents how it speaks to the customer in every Instagram caption, Web site banner and service email.

Define the "Tone of Voice Guidelines." These guidelines represent how the brand speaks. Will the voice be empathetic but not overly sweet, or scientific but not condescending.

**Visual identity** During early development of the hero product, invest in a cohesive visual identity. This does not necessarily mean expensive, but rather cohesive. This is where the brand psychology (DNA) and voice join to create a visual language. Respected brands maintain a rigorous visual consistency across every touchpoint. To this extent, almost always the brand should hire an experienced designer. Key deliverables are

- Color palette
- Typography
- Logo system

***Avoid the templates*** Step away from generic templates used by generic web design firms. In the era of artificial intelligence, and great designers available on part-time basis, this is certainly not needed. Custom typography or a highly specific, minimalist packaging structure immediately signals that this product belongs in a higher tier.

**Packaging system** In skincare, packaging is almost always the first touchpoint to the brand and thus must be your absolute best foot forward. Decide on your primary packaging (jar, tube, pump, and so forth). Secondary packaging is the outer box (folding carton). This is the billboard in retail stores and must be perfected. From an operational and logistics perspective, hiring an experienced designer to handle packaging system design is absolutely critical. Many delays in production of goods happen when packaging systems are incorrect, delayed, or inconsistent.

In 2026, skincare consumers favored brands that reflect health, discipline, scientific rigor, and substantial social proof. Successful brands utilize social media as a "digital storefront" to communicate the product's purpose and showcase verifiable before-and-after results on actual customers.

*The Ordinary:* This brand revolutionized the industry by branding "transparency" and "clinical chemistry." Their minimalist, apothecary-style packaging and naming conventions (using ingredient names like "Niacinamide 10% + Zinc 1%") created a brand identity centered on honesty. They empowered the consumer to become their own chemist, which built a massive, cult-like following. Their visual identity is unmistakable.

*La Roche-Posay:* Their brand is built on the foundation of "Thermal Spring Water" and a deep connection to the European (ie, French) dermatologic roots. By using a consistent blue-and-white clinical esthetic, they signal safety, medical-grade quality, and French pharmaceutical heritage. This branding reassures the consumer that the product is tested on even the most sensitive skin. This brand provides a great example of packaging, and visual identity.

*Topicals:* Topicals built its identity by rejecting the sterile, heavily retouched esthetic of traditional skincare in favor of "radical" authenticity. The brand utilizes its digital storefront to showcase unedited before-and-after photos of customers dealing with chronic flare-ups and hyperpigmentation. By normalizing visible skin conditions and fostering a highly engaged, vocal community, the brand positioned itself as both a scientifically rigorous treatment and an inclusive cultural movement. When it comes to mastering psychological brand identity, this company is the sine qua non.

*CeraVe:* The brand cemented its modern identity around accessibility and dermatologist-backed efficacy. By maintaining a straightforward, no-nonsense visual identity and heavily leveraging user-generated content alongside professional endorsements, CeraVe built a brand synonymous with reliable, dermatologist-recommended skincare. Their digital storefronts rely heavily on educational content directly from medical professionals, serving as the ultimate social proof.

*SkinCeuticals:* As a pioneer in antioxidant science, the brand cultivated a prestige identity centered entirely on clinical evidence and professional authority. Their branding utilizes heavy glass dropper bottles, scientific nomenclature, and a strict public adherence to peer-reviewed research. By intentionally positioning their products alongside plastic surgeons and high-end dermatologists rather than traditional retail shelves, the brand successfully signals luxury through the lens of uncompromising scientific discipline.

### *Step 5: determine product-market fit*

> *Anything that won't sell, I don't want to invent it. Its sale is proof of utility, and utility is success.*
>
> *—Thomas Edison*

Ultimately, product-market fit is determined by whether the customer agrees that the formulation solves a legitimate problem at an acceptable price—and proves it by actually spending their own money. Focus groups are often insufficient, as they are typically composed of individuals eager to please. Instead, actual purchasing behavior, or the lack thereof, serves as the most critical form of feedback.

**The Amazon Benchmark** Approximately 80% of Amazon searches are unbranded, making it a powerful tool to test if a product fills a general need. This means that a majority of searches for skin care are targeting a problem in search of a solution rather than searching for a specific brand. In effect, small brands that identify relevant skincare problems that have few solutions can become market leaders.

**Performance metrics** For the Skintensive Bruise Cream, a 20% repeat customer rate and a low 1.3% return rate indicated an excellent fit. For KP Away, a 40% repeat customer rate indicated a very strong fit despite many large brands competing for the same customer. Conversely, another brand "Siberian Silk" cream failed to find a fit, with monthly sales stagnating the brand ultimately shut down.

*Bio-Oil:* This product found perfect market fit by becoming the synonymous solution for "stretch marks and scars." Despite being a simple oil blend, its specific positioning and affordable price point led to global dominance in pharmacies. Its high repeat purchase rate among pregnant women and postsurgery patients confirms a deep market need.

*EltaMD:* This brand found its fit within the professional channel, specifically through dermatologist recommendations for daily sun protection. By formulating a sunscreen that felt like a moisturizer and did not leave a white cast (UV Clear), they solved the primary reason people avoid SPF.

## SUMMARY

The successful entrepreneur identifies a problem, develops a tangible solution, and ultimately builds a cohesive brand and a thriving business. In the early stages, focus must remain squarely on problem identification, consumer specificity, fastidious product development, and achieving product-market fit—proven the moment a customer validates the value proposition with their own money.

As demonstrated over the last 40 years by legacy names like Proactiv and Murad, and newer brands like SEEN, dermatologists are uniquely positioned to launch clinical ideas that can transform from rapid prototypes into household brands. The companies that achieve this level of success are those that prioritize reliability over fleeting trends, listen closely to their customers, and innovate rapidly.

To truly scale, founders must eventually transition from working in the business to working on it. When the founder can step away and the operations run without skipping a beat, the company is truly prepared for the long haul. Ultimately, the longevity of any young brand rests on the dedication of its founder. This path is long, demanding, and requires far more than a "side hustle" commitment—but for the clinician willing to take the leap, it is absolutely worthwhile.

## CLINICS CARE POINTS

- Define a specific market gap.
- Identify the initial specific customer.
- Detailed Product development.
- Develop and refine the brand identity.
- Collect sales data to confirm product-market fit.

## ARTIFICIAL INTELLIGENCE DECLARATION

During the preparation of this article, the authors used Gemini for Tone Calibration and ensure consistent grammar and reference citation. After using this tool/service, the author reviewed and edited the content as needed and takes full responsibility for the content of the publication.

## DISCLOSURE

A. Mikailov is the cofounder of Skintensive LLC and Boston Skin Science LLC (dba KPAway).

## REFERENCES

1. Mordor intelligence. Skin care products market size & share analysis - growth trends and forecast (2026 - 2031). Mordor intelligence. 2026. Available at: https://www.mordorintelligence.com/industry-reports/skincare-products-market. Accessed March 2, 2026.
2. Coherent Market Insights. Dermocosmetics skin care products market size and share analysis - growth trends and forecasts (2026-2033). Coherent market insights. 2025. Available at: https://www.coherentmarketinsights.com/industry-reports/dermocosmetics-skin-care-products-market. Accessed March 1, 2026.
3. Faizullabhoy M, Wani G. Dermocosmetics Market Size & Share 2024 – 2032. Global Market insights. 2025. Available at: https://www.gminsights.com/industry-analysis/dermocosmetics-market. Accessed March 1, 2026.
4. Fortune business insights. Dermocosmetics market size, share & industry analysis, by type, by distribution channel, and regional forecast, 2026-2034. Fortune business insights. 2026. Available at: https://www.fortunebusinessinsights.com/dermocosmetics-market-108947. Accessed March 11, 2026.
5. Helms workshop. "What is Brand Equity." helms workshop. Available at: https://helmsworkshop.com/blog/what-is-brand-equity. Accessed March 9, 2026.

# Branding and the Business of Dermatology

Britany Hartshorn, BS[a], Cheryl Burgess, MD, FAAD[b,*]

KEYWORDS

• Ethical medical branding • Dermatology branding • Professional development • Networking

KEY POINTS

- The visual nature of dermatology provides an avenue for professional brand development and patient engagement.
- Board-certified dermatologists have the unique opportunity to enhance the safety standards and quality of commercial skincare.
- Branding in dermatology can advance career opportunities, expand your professional network, increase access to resources, and establish you as a thought leader in your field.
- A dermatology brand should be grounded in personal interest, expertise, and values, and all brand promotion should follow the ethical principles of medical practice.

## INTRODUCTION

Dermatology occupies a unique position in medicine, with a range of therapeutic interventions that address both systemic and localized disease, enhance esthetics, and, by extension, mental well-being. This wide scope of practice and the visual nature of dermatology provide an avenue for meaningful patient and public engagement. As a result, dermatologists have the opportunity to engage in product development, cosmetic innovation, media education, and industry collaboration. However, given advancements in technology, the evolving digital landscape in medicine, and direct-to-consumer health care models, there is now an information paradox. Patients have unprecedented access to medical information at their fingertips but are simultaneously inundated with a surge in unregulated medical misinformation. Most skin care information shared online through forums and social media posts is shared by nonphysician "skinfluencers" who promote idealized skin, are motivated by brand deals and clout, and do not have the formal education to understand the active ingredients that make up the products they are promoting.[1] This creates the demand for an ethically guided and medically sound dermatology digital influence. Unlike "skinfluencers," estheticians, and other non–board-certified providers, board-certified dermatologists receive extensive formal education and training with an emphasis on evidence-based care and a commitment to patient safety. This further reinforces the unique value dermatologists bring to an increasingly crowded and commercially driven marketplace.

In this environment, professional success in dermatology depends not only on formal education and clinical excellence but also on the development of a strategic and visual identity.[2] Branding in dermatology is the creation of an intentional, professional identity grounded in values and evidence-based expertise. Creating a dermatology brand can set you apart from competitors and can serve as a public health service to combat misinformation, the promotion of

[a] Burrell College of Health Sciences, School of Osteopathic Medicine, Melbourne, FL, USA; [b] Department of Dermatology, Center for Dermatology and Dermatologic Surgery, Washington D.C, USA
* Corresponding author. 2311 M Street, Northwest, Suite 504, Washington, DC, 20037-1495.
*E-mail address:* cheryl.burgess@Ctr4dermatology.com
Twitter: @HartsBritany (B. H)

Dermatol Clin 44 (2026) 555–561
https://doi.org/10.1016/j.det.2026.06.001

| Abbreviation | |
|---|---|
| AMA | American Medical Association |

idealized skin, and harmful "*social media dysmorphia*" that can lead to unrealistic patient expectations and increased risk to skin health.[3] With an emphasis on clinical excellence and differentiation from competitors, creating a dermatology brand can establish your authority in both the online skin space, by helping to guide patients to safe and effective care, and in your professional community by establishing you as a thought leader among your colleagues. This article evaluates the benefits and ethical considerations of branding in dermatology and provides a strategic framework for dermatologists seeking to define their niche, expand their influence, build professional networks, and make an impact.

## DISCUSSION

### *Defining Branding in Dermatology*

Branding is the intentional effort to develop a unique personality that distinguishes your products or services from competitors. The *what* and the *why* of the brand should be based on your values as a clinician and should fall within your area of expertise. Branding allows patients to connect with you through shared values and personal experiences and is critical to the brand's success and credibility.[4] It tells the patient why you care and why you are a credible source, lets the patient in on the mission, and establishes rapport. In the modern medical landscape, a successful brand must have an online presence. Online visibility increases patients' and colleagues' access to and understanding of the brand, which translates into brand engagement and growth.

When defining a dermatology brand, consider how you want the brand to be interpreted and intentionally translate this into every aspect of the brand experience. Branding in dermatology is much more than a name or logo; it is the intentional curation of every aspect of the brand, from name, logo, and content to how patients and colleagues can interact with the brand. This concept is known as the "digital front door" and encompasses the different channels through which people view and interact with the brand, such as Web site user experience, social media engagement, and educational content.[5] Each aspect of your brand should reinforce its identity and provide an opportunity for meaningful engagement. When the identity of your brand is clearly and consistently communicated, it allows for the opportunity to connect with others and can provide several benefits, both personally and professionally. The advantages of branding include differentiation, professional reputation, career advancement, networking, thought leadership, personal development, and business opportunities.

### *Personal Branding and Professional Advancement*

Developing your personal brand involves self-reflection, identification of your strengths and values, and aligning them with your professional goals and aspirations. When done effectively, branding highlights your interests, knowledge base, and achievements, ultimately establishing your credibility and building trust in your brand. Beyond the clinic, a brand can diversify your career portfolio, reach of influence, and your streams of income. By positioning yourself through the creation and promotion of your brand as a niche expert, you open the doors for nonclinical opportunities such as consulting, serving on industry advisory boards, editorial positions for journals, or providing specialized expertise as a medical-legal witness, to name a few. These opportunities can help to enhance fulfillment in your career by diversifying your influence and keeping you engaged and up to date in the industry and can bring in additional streams of revenue to buffer against decreasing insurance reimbursement rates.

Brand development provides opportunities to connect and collaborate with colleagues, mentors, and industry leaders, fostering organic, meaningful connections that lead to the pooling of ideas and resources.[6] Think of brand networking and the sharing of resources as analogous to asking to borrow a cup of sugar from a neighbor. Of course, you could run to the store, but borrowing sugar from your neighbor saves time and builds community. This is referred to as "Social Capital theory." The idea behind Social Capital theory is that our lives, and therefore our professional ventures, are made more productive and, therefore, more fulfilling when we build an interconnected social network. According to Social Capital theory, the value this network holds is based on trust and reciprocity.[7] When borrowing a cup of sugar from your neighbor, you are setting the precedent for collaboration, and similarly, when building a community around your brand, you are creating a support system to help protect against burnout and open the door for pooling of ideas, sharing of resources, and exploration of insights and perspectives that can keep your brand relevant and add value. By challenging yourself to network, staying up to date within your area of expertise, and engaging with people through content creation, public speaking, or social media, you position yourself as a thought leader, gain visibility within your field, and expand your professional influence. People are more likely to engage with individuals they know, trust, and perceive as experts.

## Practical Framework for Building a Dermatology Brand

When starting, your focus should be on defining your niche and figuring out what sets you apart from others in the field. Here, we provide a structured step-by-step framework to build your own brand. These steps are intentionally identified to guide you through a successful brand creation. (1) Perform a self-assessment of core strengths and professional interests. (2) Define the patient population or professional community you want to serve. (3) Determine short-term and long-term goals. (4) Articulate what unique expertise you can provide. (5) Market your brand and raise brand awareness. (6) Audit brand health to ensure that brand messaging aligns with patient perception (Fig. 1). By first performing a self-assessment, you are able to identify potential gaps in dermatologic care that matter to you and outline how your expertise and knowledge can help to bridge the gap and provide meaningful care to patients. Defining your patient population early on will help guide the creation of your brand and the establishment of short-term and long-term goals, which will act as a roadmap and keep you centered. Long-term goals are important as they provide vision, direction, and purpose, while short-term goals allow for more immediate actions and accomplishments. There should be a re-evaluation of your brand over time, and therefore, long-term goals can change in response to the accumulation of completed short-term goals, or in response to changing needs of the professional community and/or patient population. Brand marketing, the fifth step in our proposed framework, is only possible after determining your niche and the specific expertise and services that you will provide. While marketing strategies often overlap to include social media, advertisements, public speaking, educational initiatives, and professional affiliations, regardless of the specific area of focus, the details on how you promote your brand matter and can be crucial in its perception and credibility. Here, we provide a few marketing strategy examples to consider when choosing how best to market your brand (Table 1). Finally, you must focus on brand health by remaining curious, involved, and willing to reassess brand positioning in light of evolving career goals, the changing business landscape, and patient needs.

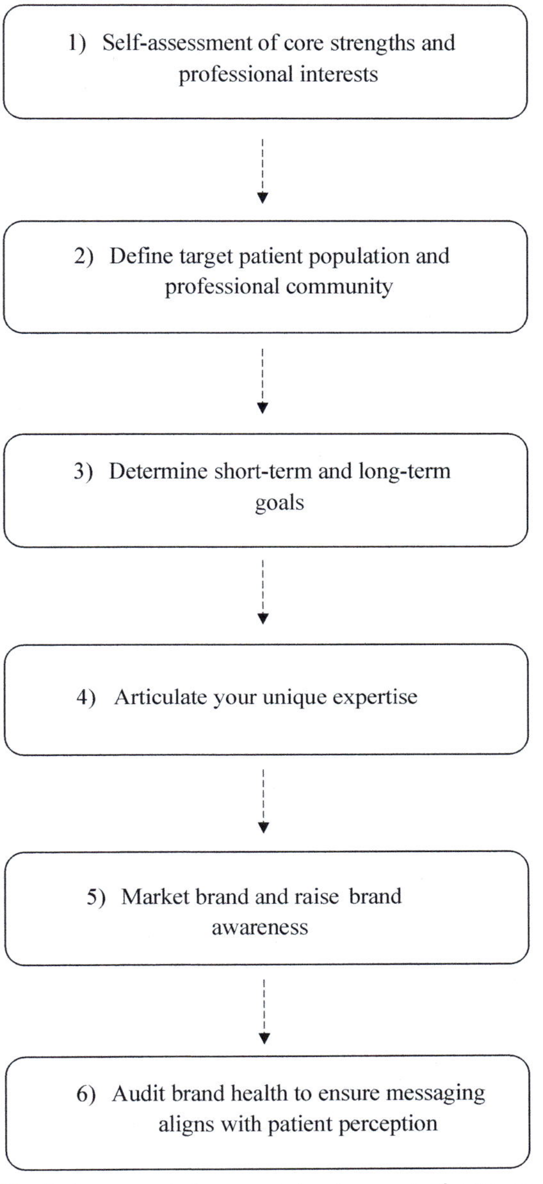


Fig. 1. Framework for brand development. The image depicts a simple 6 step framework to guide the successful development of a personal and professional brand in dermatology.

## Inclusive Branding and Product Innovation

Diversity is inherent in the practice of dermatology. Given that dermatology centers on the diagnosis and treatment of the skin, hair, and nails, dermatologists must incorporate diversity into their education and training so that they can recognize and

**Table 1**
**Niche-based marketing strategies**

| Brand Focus | Marketing Strategy | Strategic Objective |
|---|---|---|
| Medical dermatology | Attend academic conferences. Bring awareness to diseases through public speaking. Network with pharmaceutical companies for research development | Clinical authority: To stay at the forefront of emerging systemic treatments. To educate colleagues and patients |
| Esthetic dermatology | Attend esthetic-focused symposia. Teach courses on emerging techniques. Provide social media demos of services. Share consented patient testimonials | Visual credibility: To demonstrate technical proficiency and realistic patient outcomes. To educate colleagues on emerging techniques, products, and patient outcomes |
| Surgical dermatology | Publish research articles. Demonstrate surgical techniques to colleagues. Collaborate with device manufactures | Technical expertise: To highlight precision and safety in procedural outcomes. To build referring physician trust |
| Pediatric dermatology, rural dermatology, or niche subspecialties | Lead patient education workshops. Engage in advocacy through nonprofits, and multilingual patient resources | Community trust: To establish a brand as a safe and accessible resource for specific vulnerable populations. Educate patients on skin health |
| Business of cosmeceuticals | Private label formulations with science-based ingredients that are more efficacious than recommending over-the-counter products | Quality and convenience: Rather than directing patients to a drugstore, this approach allows them to purchase curated, physician-dispensed products directly from your practice |

The table provides illustrative examples of brand marketing in dermatology.

manage conditions in different skin tones and hair types. Historically, representation of skin of color has been lacking in formal medical education and in dermatology literature. This has led to lower diagnostic accuracy, decreased quality of care, poorer treatment outcomes, and negative patient experiences in patients with skin of color.[8] More recently, there have been efforts to bridge the gap not only through reformation of formal medical education but also by increasing cultural competency and humility. This same commitment to inclusivity should be reflected in the development of a dermatology brand. An inclusive brand offers a range of products or services suitable for patients of different racial and ethnic backgrounds, genders, and abilities. Brand content creation should depict this inclusivity and should be sensitive to different cultures. One way to promote inclusivity is to offer brand materials in multiple languages (eg, product packaging, social media with multilingual closed captions, and so forth).[9] Inclusive product innovation can also be driven by actively engaging with patients and listening to their feedback. Inclusivity means putting the patient's needs at the forefront of the brand and incorporating their feedback.

Building an inclusive dermatology brand extends beyond content creation, products, and services to workforce diversity and advocacy for diagnostic parity. By hiring staff that reflects a diverse range of ethnicities, races, and cultures, a brand moves beyond deploying inclusivity and diversity as a marketing tactic to being a brand that actively practices inclusion. Making inclusivity inherent to the brand can help to build brand trust and loyalty among patients who see people similar to themselves as an integral part of the brand. Dermatology can be an intimate and vulnerable experience for patients, and building a brand where they can feel seen, understood, and safe not only benefits the success of the brand but also the patient–provider relationship and ultimately patient health outcomes.

## *Rebranding in Dermatology*

Rebranding is the updating or creation of a new name, term, symbol, design, or combination thereof for an established brand, with the intention of developing a differentiated position in the minds of stakeholders and competitors. A company may consider rebranding for several reasons: to keep up with the economic landscape, such as changes in patient needs or technological advancements; to update brand values to reflect the current culture; to maintain relevance and an edge over competitors; or to support brand expansion and growth.[10] Rebranding is not without some risk, so the decision to rebrand should be made only after a careful analysis of the demands placed on the brand, where the brand currently stands, and a detailed plan for future projections. A successful rebrand would include aligning the company's image with updated values and goals while retaining the previous patient base and expanding and gaining new patients. Companies that have successfully rebranded have done so using an inside-out approach, evaluating internal areas of improvement and making changes patiently over time while avoiding radical changes to the brand name or logo. A famous example of this was Apple's late 1990s rebranding, where they simplified their brand and focused on the user experience.[11] For a dermatologist, this translates into focusing on the patient experience. To rebrand, the company must re-evaluate all aspects of the patient experience from the clinic to product and digital communications to ensure that the patient experience is in alignment with the brand's values and purpose.

Preservation of name and logo is not always possible, especially with company mergers or when the original name and logo were too niche, outdated, or no longer accurately representing the direction in which the brand has grown. In instances like this, there should be an effort to maintain brand equity, or the recognizable aspects of the brand that patients have come to know and trust. For example, if the logo must be changed, a brand can use the same color palette for the new logo to enhance patient recognition, or when undergoing a merger, keep the same company staff, especially during the period of transition. This will preserve the human experience of your brand even when new names or logos might not yet be familiar. By honoring these familiar elements, a brand can communicate that there has not been a loss of identity but rather a continued commitment to a more inclusive future for its patients.

## *Ethical Considerations*

Ethical considerations regarding branding in dermatology are an important and popular topic of discussion. A study published in November 2025 surveyed members of the American Academy of Dermatology and brought to light some recurring ethical dilemmas shared by dermatologists. Dilemmas mentioned in the study include financial influence and related conflicts of interest and their potential effect on quality of care and provider decision-making, overuse of procedures and or products for financial gain, and misrepresentation of provider qualifications/scope of practice.[12] Before diving further into a discussion of medical ethics, it is important to note that, according to the American Medical Association's (AMA) Code of Medical Ethics on Advertising & Publicity, physicians may promote themselves (and, by extension, their brand) through any form of public communication, provided the information is truthful and does not mislead or deceive.[13]

The provided ethical dos and don'ts chart (**Table 2**) is not all-encompassing but instead is meant to engage you in thought as you create, navigate, and promote an ethical dermatology brand. This chart addresses 6 ethical areas of concern shared among dermatologists regarding the promotion of products and services, with the first being public communication. All forms of communication from a brand, whether that be product packaging, social media posts, or public speaking events, should be truthful and evidence-based, should not be meant to deceive the reasonable patient, and, to the best of its ability, should avoid setting a precedent of unrealistic expectations. This commitment to honesty should extend to financial influence in that the brand should not recommend products or perform services purely in the spirit of increasing procedural volume and therefore financial gain. All products and services should be decided on collaboratively with patients and should be made in the best interest of the patient. Furthermore, any financial conflicts of interest should be disclosed, and physicians should accurately represent their specific credentials and avoid performing services or offering advice outside of their training. Finally, the chart emphasizes that a truly ethical brand should incorporate inclusivity by actively listening to and addressing the specific needs of diverse patient populations as a commitment to diagnostic parity and equitable care. Ultimately, brand promotion and financial gain should not be valued over clinical integrity. When creating and promoting a brand, one should approach every decision in alignment with a commitment to act in the best interest of the patient, to do no harm, and to only offer services, products, and/or procedures that are evidence-based and that are a medically sound option for the patient.

**Table 2**
**Ethical considerations and best practices for branding in dermatology**

| Feature | The "Dos" (Ethical Best Practices) | The "Don'ts" (Ethical Pitfalls) |
|---|---|---|
| Public communication | Ensure all promotional information is truthful and evidence-based[13] | Avoid any communication that could mislead or deceive a reasonable patient[13] |
| Financial influence | Disclose potential conflicts of interest regarding product development or industry ties[12] | Never allow financial incentives to dictate provider decision-making or quality of care[12] |
| Inclusivity | Recommend treatments only when clinically indicated for the patient's well-being | Avoid the overuse of procedures or products driven primarily by financial gain |
| Procedure volume | Clearly and accurately represent your specific qualifications and training[12] | Do not misrepresent your scope of practice or credentials[12] |
| Professional scope | Act in the best interest of the patient at all times (Beneficence) | Avoid offering services, procedures, or products that are not evidence-based |
| Patient interests | Incorporate inclusive innovation by listening to feedback from diverse patient populations[9] | Do not exclude or ignore specific needs of a diverse patient population[9] |

This chart contrasts "Dos" and "Don'ts," based on the AMA Code of Ethics, to guide clinicians in maintaining professional integrity in brand development and promotion.

## SUMMARY

In the current day and age, branding in medicine and providing a visible way for patients and leaders in the field to experience and connect with your brand is more important than ever. With advances in technology and information at patients' fingertips, it is increasingly important to educate patients and promote evidence-based medicine they can trust. In this article, we provide a practical 6 step framework to guide you in your brand development, define branding and rebranding, highlight the benefits of branding, such as personal and professional advancement, discuss important ethical considerations, and recommend tips for brand success, such as inclusivity, a willingness to re-evaluate the brand often, and consideration of patient feedback for brand improvement.

## CLINICS CARE POINTS

- *Pearl*: Successful branding should be an intentional extension of your values and specific areas of expertise. Aligning your professional personality with your clinical strengths establishes rapport.
- *Pearl*: Engagement in networking, education, research, and public communication can enhance brand visibility, strengthen brand credibility, and establish thought leadership.
- *Pearl*: Per the AMA's ethics of clinical practice, dermatologists may engage in self-promotion and professional branding, provided they are truthful, within their scope of practice, do not cause harm, and align with ethical standards.
- *Pearl*: Ensure that any products or procedures promoted are strictly evidence-based and that the patient's best interests are prioritized over financial gain.
- *Pitfall*: Neglecting brand inclusivity (eg, packaging, digital content, and products/services) and patient feedback.
- *Pitfall*: Unwillingness to re-evaluate the brand in light of patient feedback and the ever-changing landscape of medicine.

## DISCLOSURE

C. Burgess is a cofounder of Black Opal and serves as a consultant for RoC, SkinMedica, and IT Cosmetics. All other authors report no relevant financial conflicts of interest.

## REFERENCES

1. Werpachowski N, Adebiyi O, Edupuganti N, et al. Establishing physician-governed social media accreditation to combat the spread of misinformation by non-medical skinfluencers. Dermis 2025;5(5). https://doi.org/10.35702/derm.10049.

2. Seyferth AV, Egan JM, Chung KC. Branding in health care. Plast Reconstr Surg 2022;150(3):481–5.
3. Frasier K, Werpachowski N, Hash MG, et al. Chasing digital perfection in a filtered world: the role of dermatologists in addressing social media dysmorphia. J Cosmet Dermatol 2026;25(1):e70672.
4. Ackovska A, Grozdanova A, Sterjev Z, et al. The role of branding in the healthcare system with special review to healthcare institutions. Knowl Int J 2020; 41(3):489–94.
5. Rastogi N. Healthcare's new frontier: the digital front door. BMJ Innov 2022;8(2):129–32.
6. Jenssen JI, Koenig HF. The effect of social networks on resource access and business start-ups. Eur Plan Stud 2002;10(8):1039–46.
7. Putnam R. Bowling alone: the collapse and revival of American community. New York (NY): Simon & Schuster Paperbacks; 2000.
8. Syder NC, Omar D, McKenzie S, et al. Gaps in medical education curricula on skin of color in medical school, residency, and beyond: part 1. J Am Acad Dermatol 2023;89(5):885–92.
9. Verbytska A, Lysenko I, Babachenko L, et al. Inclusive social marketing: representation and diversity in brand campaigns. Marketing and Branding Research 2023;10:45–58.
10. Goi CL, Goi MT. Review on models and reasons of rebranding. In: proceedings of the international conference on social science and humanityVol 5. Singapore: IACSIT Press; 2011. p. V2-445–2-449.
11. Todor RD. The importance of branding and rebranding for strategic marketing. Bull Transilv Univ Brasov Ser V Econ Sci 2014;7(2):59.
12. Huang C, Sangari A, Sood A, et al. Ethical dilemmas in clinical dermatology: a qualitative analysis of American Academy of Dermatology Member Survey responses. J Clin Aesthet Dermatol 2025;18(11): 30–6.
13. American Medical Association. American Medical Association AMA code of ethics. 1847. Available at: https://policysearch.ama-assn.org/policyfinder/detail/Advertising%20and%20publicity?uri=%2FAMADoc%2FEthics.xml-E-9.6.1.xml. Accessed April 5, 2026.

# Developing a Dermatology-Specific Electronic Medical Record

## Leadership, Strategy, and the Role of Artificial Intelligence

Srdjan Prodanovich, MD, FAAD

**KEYWORDS**

- Dermatology EHR • Clinical workflow • Physician leadership • Artificial intelligence
- Health technology • Specialty-specific systems

**KEY POINTS**

- Dermatology presents unique clinical, procedural, and longitudinal documentation challenges that are poorly served by generic electronic medical record systems.
- Physician-led design is essential for translating dermatologic workflows into useable, clinically meaningful digital platforms.
- Specialty-specific electronic medical records provide the foundation for meaningful integration of artificial intelligence in dermatology.
- Artificial intelligence in dermatology must be multimodal, specialty-aware, and embedded within structured clinical data to improve care quality while reducing physician burden.

## INTRODUCTION

Electronic medical records (EHRs) have become ubiquitous in modern medicine, yet their promise of improved efficiency and care coordination remains unevenly realized. While many specialties have adapted—sometimes begrudgingly—to generalized EHR platforms, dermatology continues to experience a disproportionate mismatch between clinical workflow and EHR design. This mismatch is not merely an inconvenience; it has meaningful consequences for patient care, physician satisfaction, and the accuracy, consistency, and longitudinal usability of clinical data.

Dermatology is a high-volume, visually driven specialty that relies heavily on pattern recognition, longitudinal follow-up, and procedural documentation. A single patient encounter may involve the evaluation of multiple, diverse dermatologic conditions, including inflammatory dermatoses and numerous lesions, each with distinct morphologies, anatomic locations, and management decisions. Dermatologic decision-making routinely integrates clinical photography, dermoscopy, dermatopathologic findings, and comparison across prior encounters. Generic EHR systems, largely designed for text-based documentation and problem-oriented medical encounters, are not optimized to support this level of visual and procedural complexity and may disrupt, rather than complement, dermatologic workflow.

As regulatory demands, documentation requirements, and administrative burdens continue to expand, dermatologists increasingly find themselves spending more time interacting with software rather than with patients. Burnout, now recognized as a systemic issue in medicine, is exacerbated when digital tools fail to align with clinical reality.[1] Addressing this challenge requires more than incremental optimization of existing systems;

Advanced Dermatologic and Cosmetic Institute, 90 Cypress Way E, Suite 50, Naples, FL 34110, USA
*E-mail address:* info@drprodanovich.com

Dermatol Clin 44 (2026) 563–570
https://doi.org/10.1016/j.det.2026.05.002
0733-8635/26/

**Abbreviations**

| | |
|---|---|
| AI | artificial intelligence |
| UX | user experience |

it requires rethinking how EHRs are designed, led, and implemented within dermatology.

Moreover, as artificial intelligence (AI) becomes increasingly integrated into clinical medicine, the limitations of generalized EHR architectures extend beyond workflow inefficiency to the quality and structure of the data that will ultimately shape future diagnostic and decision-support tools.

## IDENTIFYING THE GAP IN DERMATOLOGY EHRs

### *Documentation Complexity in Real-world Practice*

Dermatology encounters are often highly information-dense. Unlike many specialties in which a visit may focus on a single problem over an extended period, dermatologists frequently address multiple, unrelated conditions across all age groups within a single, time-limited encounter—ranging from benign lesions and inflammatory dermatoses to premalignant and malignant neoplasms. Each condition may require a distinct assessment, procedural intervention, patient counseling, and individualized follow-up plan.

Generic EHRs typically force this complexity into linear, problem-based notes or free-text narratives. While flexible, free-text documentation undermines consistency, complicates retrieval of prior clinical data, and limits downstream usability. This limitation is particularly pronounced in dermatology, a specialty with a highly developed descriptive language and specialized terminology used to convey morphology, distribution, texture, and pattern. Dermatology encompasses thousands of distinct conditions, an extensive morphologic vocabulary, and highly granular anatomic descriptors, making purely narrative documentation difficult to standardize, retrieve, and analyze longitudinally—particularly in high-volume practices where documentation is frequently distributed across scribes or ancillary team members who may not share the same depth of dermatologic training. As a result, identifying how a specific lesion has evolved over time becomes challenging when prior descriptions are buried in narrative notes rather than captured as structured, searchable data.[2]

### *Coding Challenges: ICD-10 versus SNOMED-CT*

The disconnect between clinical reasoning and billing systems is particularly evident in dermatology. Dermatologists conceptualize disease in terms of morphology, distribution, and dermatopathologic correlation—elements that are well represented in clinical terminologies such as SNOMED-CT, a comprehensive, multilingual clinical health care terminology collection maintained by an international nonprofit standards development organization. In contrast, reimbursement and reporting rely on international classification of diseases, tenth revision (ICD-10) codes, which often lack the granularity necessary to fully capture dermatologic nuance.

Generic EHR platforms frequently require clinicians to select billing codes directly, thereby forcing the real-time translation of clinically intuitive documentation into complex, frequently revised administrative coding frameworks. Notably, some platforms marketed as dermatology-specific retain this same underlying architecture, resulting in similar documentation and coding inefficiencies despite specialty branding.

In high-volume dermatology practices, this documentation burden is often distributed across scribes or ancillary staff to maintain clinic throughput, a workflow that can introduce additional opportunities for transcription error or misalignment between clinical intent and recorded data. These inefficiencies may propagate downstream, increasing the risk of inaccurate coding, delayed billing, and data inconsistency. A dermatology-specific EHR can instead allow clinicians to document care using clinically meaningful terminology while automating the conversion to appropriate billing codes in the background, thereby preserving accuracy, efficiency, and data fidelity.

### *Procedures, Biopsies, and Body Mapping*

Procedural care is central to dermatology. Biopsies, excisions, cryotherapy, photodynamic therapy, laser treatments, and cosmetic procedures are routine components of daily practice. Accurate documentation requires precise anatomic localization—often down to subcentimeter resolution—which is essential for both clinical decision-making and accurate procedural coding. Moreover, dermatologic care is inherently longitudinal; individual lesions are monitored over months or years, and even subtle changes—or misidentification of lesion location—may carry significant clinical implications.[3]

In addition to its clinical importance, precise anatomic localization is frequently required for accurate procedural coding. Many dermatologic current procedural terminology (CPT) codes are site-specific, such that the same procedure—such as a biopsy or excision—may be coded differently depending on whether it is performed on the eyelid margin, cheek, ear, or other anatomically distinct regions. Imprecise documentation of lesion location, therefore, has downstream consequences for coding accuracy and administrative efficiency.

Electronic health records (EHR) systems employ varying approaches to anatomic documentation; however, 2 dimensional body mapping remains the most common. While sufficient for basic notation, 2 dimensional mapping introduces inherent limitations when applied to the 3 dimensional surface of the human body. Accurately documenting a single lesion may require multiple 2 dimensional views to approximate depth, curvature, and spatial relationships, increasing documentation burden and interuser variability.

An instructive analogy is navigation using multiple static paper maps to traverse long distances, compared with modern Global Positioning System-based systems that dynamically track precise location in 3 dimensional space. Similarly, 2 dimensional body maps often fail to preserve exact lesion location over time, limiting reliable lesion reidentification and accurate anatomic comparison during follow-up visits.

A 3 dimensional body mapping approach addresses these limitations by providing sufficient anatomic granularity to support efficient documentation at the point of care. When precise anatomic locations are selected directly within a 3 dimensional representation, biopsy and procedural details can be captured accurately during the encounter, enabling appropriate CPT code selection without reliance on post hoc interpretation of narrative descriptions. This integration reduces ambiguity, improves efficiency, and supports both clinical accuracy and downstream administrative workflows.

As a result, dermatologists are less reliant on external systems, scanned drawings, or disconnected imaging platforms to supplement documentation. Reducing this fragmentation helps preserve workflow continuity and enables the creation of cohesive longitudinal datasets essential for high-quality patient care, outcomes tracking, and future analytical and AI applications.[4]

## PHYSICIAN-LED PRODUCT DEVELOPMENT

### *Why Dermatologists Must Lead Design*

Many shortcomings of existing EHRs can be traced to their origins as systems designed primarily by technologists or administrators with limited exposure to daily clinical practice. In many cases, contemporary platforms are built on legacy architectures originally developed for other medical specialties, thereby constraining flexibility and limiting their ability to accommodate the workflow-intensive demands unique to dermatology. Additional pressures to prioritize scalability, standardization, and financial performance—often driven by organizational or ownership structures—can further shift emphasis away from usability and clinician-centered design.

As a result, product development and implementation are frequently guided by individuals with deep technical or operational expertise but limited medical or dermatologic training. This structural disconnect helps explain why even systems marketed as dermatology-focused may continue to reproduce the same documentation, workflow, and usability challenges observed in generalized EHR platforms.

Dermatology-specific EHR development, and EHR design more broadly, therefore demands meaningful leadership from dermatologists who understand not only what must be documented but also how clinicians think, prioritize, and make real-time decisions in high-volume clinical environments. Physician-led design ensures that software supports clinical reasoning rather than obstructing it. Dermatologists are uniquely positioned to determine which data elements are essential, which are redundant, and which workflows must remain flexible—insight that cannot be fully captured through focus groups or post hoc feedback, but instead requires direct and sustained clinical involvement.

### *Translating Clinical Workflow into Software Logic*

Effective EHR design requires abstraction—the distillation of complex clinical processes into structured, repeatable workflows without oversimplifying them. For example, documenting a skin lesion involves capturing morphology, color, size, anatomic location, differential diagnosis, and management plan. Structuring these elements enables consistency, data reuse, and longitudinal comparison while preserving clinical nuance.

Physician-led teams are uniquely positioned to guide this translation. They can ensure that structured data entry aligns naturally with clinical thought processes rather than feeling imposed or artificial, reflecting how dermatologists examine patients and reason through skin disease in real time.

### *Avoiding Feature Bloat*

A common failure mode in health technology is feature bloat—the accumulation of infrequently used tools that clutter interfaces, slow performance, and increase cognitive load. Physician leaders are often more disciplined in resisting unnecessary complexity, prioritizing usability, speed, and clarity over exhaustive functionality.

In dermatology, where patient volume is high and visit time is limited, a streamlined design is not merely a convenience but a prerequisite for safe and efficient care delivery. Thoughtful feature selection ensures that technology enhances, rather than hinders, clinical workflow.

## STRATEGIC DECISIONS IN BUILDING A DERMATOLOGY-SPECIFIC EHR

### *Specialty Focus versus Horizontal Platforms*

A foundational strategic decision in EHR development is whether to pursue a horizontal platform designed to serve multiple medical specialties or a specialty-specific system optimized for a single domain. Horizontal EHR platforms offer advantages in scale, interoperability, and enterprise deployment, particularly within large health systems. However, these benefits are often achieved by prioritizing standardization over depth, resulting in workflows that reflect linear, problem-oriented documentation models common to many medical specialties, rather than the multidimensional, procedure-intensive, and visually driven workflows characteristic of dermatology.

Dermatology-specific EHRs adopt a fundamentally different strategic posture. Rather than attempting to accommodate all specialties equally, they prioritize depth within a single domain, enabling tighter alignment with dermatologic workflows. This includes native support for image-centric documentation, lesion-level tracking, precise anatomic localization, procedure-heavy encounters, and longitudinal follow-up. While horizontal platforms may approximate these capabilities through layered customization, such adaptations are frequently constrained by underlying architectures that were not designed for dermatology. As a result, customization on top of general-purpose systems rarely achieves the coherence, efficiency, or usability of purpose-built solutions.

From a strategic perspective, specialization represents a deliberate focus. In dermatology, where clinical nuance and efficiency are paramount, depth often delivers greater value than broad applicability.

### *Customization versus Standardization*

Another central strategic tension in EHR development is the balance between customization and standardization. Excessive customization can undermine scalability, complicate maintenance, and impair interoperability, while rigid standardization may fail to accommodate the variability inherent in real-world clinical practice.

An effective approach to dermatology-specific EHR design resolves this tension by standardizing data structures rather than clinical workflows. Core clinical elements—such as lesion morphology, anatomic location, diagnosis, procedure type, and outcome—are captured in consistent, structured formats that support mapping to standardized clinical terminologies, such as systematized nomenclature of medicine clinical terms (SNOMED-CT), thereby enabling reporting, analytics, and interoperability. At the same time, clinicians retain flexibility in how they document encounters, sequence tasks, and adapt workflows to individual practice styles.

This approach preserves structured data while allowing flexibility in clinical workflows and ensuring that documentation remains useable for longitudinal care and downstream applications, such as AI.

### *User Experience as a Strategic Asset*

User experience (UX) is often treated as a secondary consideration in health care technology, yet it plays a central role in adoption, satisfaction, and long-term viability. In dermatology, where encounters are time-limited and cognitively dense, UX is not merely a design preference but a strategic asset—particularly in environments in which documentation and workflow tasks are shared among physicians, scribes, medical assistants, and other ancillary staff.

Efficient navigation, rapid image access, minimal clicks, and intuitive data entry directly affect clinical throughput and cognitive load. Poor UX increases documentation time, fragments attention, and contributes to burnout, especially when interfaces are difficult to learn or inconsistent across user roles. Conversely, systems that align naturally with dermatologic workflows enable both clinicians and ancillary team members to perform tasks accurately and efficiently, allowing physicians to focus on patient care rather than interface management.

Strategically, investment in UX yields compounding returns. Intuitive platforms for all members of the dermatology team become embedded in daily practice, fostering adoption, consistency, and reduced attrition. In a competitive EHR market, usability across diverse user roles becomes a key differentiator, often outweighing feature breadth or technical sophistication.

### *Interoperability, Compliance, and Scalability*

Specialty-specific focus does not obviate interoperability. Dermatology EHRs must integrate seamlessly with pathology laboratories, imaging systems, referral networks, and health information exchanges. Regulatory requirements related to privacy, security, and data sharing must also be addressed proactively.

The strategic challenge lies in achieving interoperability without sacrificing usability. Overly burdensome compliance layers can erode workflow efficiency, while insufficient integration can isolate practices and limit continuity of care. Thoughtful system design ensures that regulatory and interoperability requirements are met in ways that are largely invisible to clinicians, preserving efficiency while maintaining compliance.

Scalability presents a parallel challenge. As practices grow or integrate into larger systems, EHR platforms must support increased volume, additional users, and evolving regulatory demands without degrading performance or usability. Strategic leadership is required to ensure that growth does not dilute specialty focus or compromise the clinician experience.

### *Strategic Alignment with Practice Operations*

Finally, the EHR strategy must align with the operational realities of dermatology practice. High patient volume, procedure-heavy encounters, and precise coding requirements place unique demands on both clinical and administrative workflows. Systems that separate clinical documentation from practice management functions often introduce inefficiencies, errors, and redundant data entry.

Strategically integrated platforms—those that align clinical documentation, coding logic, and operational workflows—enable practices to function more efficiently while preserving clinical accuracy. This alignment supports not only day-to-day operations but also long-term sustainability in an increasingly complex health care environment.

### *Strategic Implications*

Taken together, these strategic decisions—specialty focus, data standardization, UX prioritization, interoperability, and operational alignment—define the success or failure of dermatology-specific EHR platforms. Leadership that recognizes and navigates these trade-offs deliberately is essential to the design of systems that serve both clinicians and patients effectively.

## BRANDING AND MARKET ADOPTION

The EHR marketplace is highly saturated, with many platforms competing on feature breadth, enterprise reach, or compliance credentials. In such an environment, differentiation based solely on technical capability is increasingly difficult. For dermatology-specific platforms, meaningful differentiation arises from depth rather than breadth—specifically, from the ability to support the specialty's unique clinical, procedural, and documentation demands.

Workflow alignment represents a primary differentiator. Platforms that reduce friction, minimize redundant data entry, and support efficient navigation during time-limited encounters offer tangible value to clinicians. Similarly, native support for dermatologic imaging, anatomic precision, and longitudinal lesion tracking distinguishes specialty-focused systems from generalized alternatives.

Equally important is the ability to articulate these advantages clearly and honestly. Effective market adoption depends on transparent communication that sets realistic expectations and emphasizes clinical relevance over marketing claims. Overpromising efficiency gains or underestimating implementation complexity can erode trust and hinder adoption, particularly in a specialty that values precision and pragmatism.

### *Scaling While Preserving Identity*

Growth presents a distinct challenge for specialty-specific EHR platforms. As adoption increases, pressures often emerge to generalize functionality, broaden target markets, or standardize workflows to accommodate diverse practice settings. While such strategies may facilitate scale, they risk diluting the very characteristics that initially differentiated the platform.

Successful dermatology-specific platforms resist this tendency by preserving their core identity even as they expand. This includes maintaining a focus on dermatologic workflows, protecting usability gains achieved through specialty alignment, and avoiding design compromises that prioritize universality over relevance. Strategic scaling entails expanding capacity and interoperability without compromising the principles that made the platform effective for its primary users.

Preserving a specialty's identity also supports its long-term relevance. As health care technology continues to evolve, platforms that remain anchored in the needs of their core clinical audience are better positioned to adapt thoughtfully to new requirements, including regulatory changes and emerging technologies such as AI. Branding, trust, and adoption are tightly interwoven, shaping both initial uptake and sustained engagement.

### *Strategic Implications*

Taken together, branding and market adoption in dermatology EHRs are driven less by traditional marketing strategies than by sustained clinical alignment. Trust, differentiation, and scalability emerge from a shared foundation: respect for the specialty's complexity and a commitment to supporting dermatologists in delivering high-quality care. Platforms that recognize branding as an extension of clinical philosophy—rather than a separate commercial exercise—are more likely to achieve sustained adoption in a crowded and rapidly evolving marketplace.

### *Implementation and Sustained Engagement*

Adoption is also influenced by implementation experience. Platforms that minimize training burden, reduce disruption during onboarding, and align early with established workflows are more likely to sustain adoption. In dermatology practices—where efficiency and throughput are closely linked to financial sustainability, and institutional factors often drive adoption decisions—usability plays a critical role in long-term clinician engagement and retention.

## ARTIFICIAL INTELLIGENCE IN DERMATOLOGY EHRs

### *Why Artificial Intelligence Must Be Specialty-aware*

AI has shown promise across medicine, yet many currently deployed AI tools remain narrow and task-specific, often optimized for isolated use cases such as documentation assistance or single-image classification rather than clinical reasoning. Dermatology, by contrast, requires AI systems capable of integrating multiple data modalities—including clinical photographs, dermoscopy, dermatopathology, total-body photography, and longitudinal clinical data—within real-world workflows. Early research demonstrated the feasibility of AI-assisted differential diagnosis using clinical images alone.[5]

Recent peer-reviewed study provides compelling evidence that specialty-specific, multimodal AI architectures are better suited to these demands. In a large *Nature Medicine* study, Ge and colleagues[6] introduced a multimodal dermatology foundation model trained on more than 2 million real-world dermatologic images spanning 4 imaging modalities and multiple international institutions. The model was evaluated across diverse clinical benchmarks, including melanoma screening, differential diagnosis, lesion segmentation, longitudinal change detection, and risk stratification. Across these tasks, it consistently outperformed generalist and unimodal AI systems.

Importantly, the model demonstrated particular strength in tasks that mirror routine dermatologic practice, including longitudinal lesion monitoring, total-body photography–based risk stratification, and early melanoma detection. In reader studies, the use of the model improved clinicians' diagnostic accuracy in skin cancer assessment and enhanced differential diagnosis across a broad range of inflammatory and neoplastic conditions, with especially pronounced benefits among nonspecialist providers. Collectively, these findings underscore a critical principle: AI systems trained on dermatology-specific, multimodal, and longitudinal data are better aligned with the realities of clinical dermatology than generalist models adapted post hoc.

### *From Free Text to Structured Clinical Intelligence*

The performance gains observed in multimodal dermatology-specific AI systems are inseparable from the quality and structure of the data on which they are trained. Free-text documentation, while flexible and expressive, limits machine interpretability, reuse, and longitudinal analysis. In contrast, structured capture of key dermatologic elements—such as lesion morphology, anatomic location, diagnostic category, procedural details, and outcomes—enables AI systems to learn clinically meaningful representations that generalize across tasks.

Dermatology-specific EHRs play a foundational role in this process. By capturing clinical data in structured formats aligned with dermatologic workflows, these systems create datasets that support not only documentation and billing but also advanced analytics and AI-driven insights. The ability to link multimodal images with precise anatomic localization and longitudinal follow-up is particularly critical for tasks such as lesion change detection, risk stratification, and outcome prediction—capabilities highlighted as strengths in recent multimodal foundation models.[6]

### *Limitations of Documentation-centered Artificial Intelligence*

Much of the current clinical adoption of AI has focused on documentation assistance, including AI-based scribing and automated note generation. While these tools are relatively straightforward to implement and may offer incremental efficiency gains, they primarily operate on unstructured narrative text and do not fundamentally alter how clinical data are captured, organized, or reused.

In dermatology, where diagnostic reasoning depends on visual patterns, anatomic precision, and longitudinal change, documentation-centered AI addresses only a small fraction of the specialty's informational complexity. As a result, AI implementations limited to documentation support are insufficient to realize the broader clinical value of

AI in dermatology, which depends on structured, multimodal, and spatially precise data captured at the point of care.

### *Artificial Intelligence as a Clinical Partner*

The goal of AI in dermatology is augmentation rather than replacement.[7] AI systems are most valuable when they support clinicians' strengths—such as pattern recognition and synthesis of complex information—while reducing cognitive load and administrative burden. In reader studies, dermatology-specific AI assistance improved diagnostic accuracy and confidence without supplanting clinician judgment, illustrating a collaborative model in which clinicians retain decision-making authority while benefiting from computational support.

Crucially, effective AI must be embedded within existing clinical workflows rather than introduced as a parallel system. AI tools that require separate interfaces, duplicate data entry, or post hoc analysis risk adding friction rather than reducing it. Integration within the EHR—where clinical data, images, and longitudinal context already reside—allows AI insights to surface at the point of care, when they are most actionable.

### *Reducing Burnout through Thoughtful Integration*

When implemented thoughtfully, AI has the potential to reduce documentation burden, streamline workflows, and mitigate burnout. However, poorly designed AI—particularly systems that generate excessive alerts, provide opaque recommendations, or impose additional data-entry requirements—may exacerbate clinician fatigue. The distinction lies not in the presence of AI, but in how it is designed, governed, and integrated.

Leadership is, therefore, essential to ensure that AI serves clinicians rather than administrative metrics. Specialty-aware EHRs that prioritize structured data capture, workflow alignment, and clinician oversight provide the necessary substrate for AI systems that enhance care without undermining professional autonomy.

## LEADERSHIP CHALLENGES AND LESSONS LEARNED

### *Managing Growth and Complexity*

Developing and sustaining a dermatology-specific EHR requires navigating technical, regulatory, and organizational complexity. Growth must be managed deliberately to avoid compromising usability or trust.

### *Balancing Clinical Practice and Innovation*

Physician leaders often straddle clinical practice and technology development. Maintaining clinical involvement ensures relevance but requires disciplined prioritization and delegation.

### *Ethical and Regulatory Responsibility*

As EHRs and AI systems increasingly influence clinical decisions, ethical considerations become paramount. Transparency, data privacy, and clinician oversight must guide innovation.

## FUTURE DIRECTIONS AND IMPLICATIONS

The future of dermatology EHRs lies in deeper integration of structured data, multimodal imaging, and AI. These systems will increasingly support not only documentation but also clinical decision-making, research, and population health initiatives.

### *Implications for Training, Research, and Health Systems*

Dermatology-specific EHRs may play a growing role in education and research, enabling residents to learn from structured case libraries and supporting large-scale outcomes analysis. Health systems that invest in specialty-aware platforms may gain advantages in quality, efficiency, and innovation.

## SUMMARY

Dermatology's unique demands require digital tools designed specifically for the specialty. Physician-led development of dermatology-specific EHRs addresses long-standing gaps in workflow, documentation, and data quality. As AI advances, these platforms will serve as the foundation for meaningful innovation. Leadership, vision, and specialty focus will determine how effectively dermatology navigates the digital future.

## CLINICS CARE POINTS

Pearls

- Specialty-specific EHRs align more closely with dermatologic workflows, improving efficiency and accuracy.
- Physician leadership is essential for designing clinically meaningful digital systems.
- AI is most effective when built on structured, specialty-specific data.

Pitfalls

- Overgeneralized EHR platforms increase documentation burden and limit the utility of data.

- Poorly integrated AI tools may worsen burnout rather than alleviate it.
- Treating AI primarily as a scribe, administrative, or billing tool risks undermining its broader clinical potential.

## DISCLOSURE

S. Prodanovich reports a financial interest as the founder and creator of EZDERM, LLC.

## REFERENCES


1. Sinsky C, Colligan L, Li L, et al. Allocation of physician time in ambulatory practice: a time and motion study. Ann Intern Med 2016;165(11):753–60.
2. Altamura D, Avramidis M, Menzies SW. Assessment of the optimal interval for and sensitivity of short-term sequential digital dermoscopy monitoring for the diagnosis of melanoma. Arch Dermatol 2008;144(4):502–6.
3. Kittler H, Pehamberger H, Wolff K, et al. Diagnostic accuracy of dermoscopy. Lancet Oncol 2002;3(3):159–65.
4. Olsen CM, Primiero CA. Risk stratification for melanoma using total-body photography: a prospective cohort study. J Natl Cancer Inst 2018;110(10):1075–83.
5. Liu Y, Jain A, Eng C, et al. A deep learning system for differential diagnosis of skin diseases. Nat Med 2020;26(6):900–8.
6. Ge Z, Yan S, Yu Z, et al. A multimodal vision foundation model for clinical dermatology. Nat Med 2025;31(8):2691–702.
7. Topol EJ. High-performance medicine: the convergence of human and artificial intelligence. Nat Med 2019;25(1):44–56.

# Branding in Dermatology
## A Strategic Framework and the American Academy of Dermatology Rebranding Experience

Yiwen Helen Li, MD, MS[a], Melanie Hall, BSJ[b], Megan Cronin, MD, FAAD[c,*]

**KEYWORDS**

• Dermatology • Branding • Professional identity • Medical societies • Advocacy • Education • Innovation

**KEY POINTS**

- Branding in health care includes the expression of organizational identity—the means through which an institution communicates what is central and distinctive about its mission.
- Beyond visual identity, branding conveys purpose, signals credibility, and aligns internal culture with external perception.
- In professional medical organizations, it contributes to institutional legitimacy by shaping how stakeholders—members, patients, policymakers, and the broader public—interpret authority, relevance, and trust.

## INTRODUCTION

Branding in health care can be understood as the expression of organizational identity—the means through which an institution communicates what is central, distinctive, and enduring about its mission and role (**Fig. 1**).[1,2] Beyond visual identity, branding conveys purpose, signals credibility, and aligns internal culture with external perception.[2] In professional medical organizations, it also contributes to institutional legitimacy by shaping how stakeholders—members, patients, policymakers, and the broader public—interpret authority, relevance, and trust.[3,4]

Within dermatology, branding carries particular importance in shaping how the specialty is perceived by internal and external stakeholders. Professional organizations communicate a coherent identity while sustaining credibility within the health care system. In this context, branding contributes to both external perception and internal alignment, reinforcing shared purpose and professional identity among members.

The American Academy of Dermatology (AAD), founded in 1938, has long served as a central institutional voice in dermatology. Its identity has evolved alongside the specialty; however, the visual and narrative framework in place prior to the recent rebranding dated to 1992.[5] In the decades that followed, the practice and communication of dermatology changed substantially, shaped by the rise of digital platforms, new modes of clinical delivery, and evolving approaches to education and professional engagement. These developments contributed to a divergence between the organization's established identity and contemporary expectations, prompting the need for a revised framework capable of integrating historical continuity with forward-looking relevance.

[a] Department of Dermatology, Emory University School of Medicine, Atlanta, GA, USA; [b] Growth, Brand & Partnerships, Communication & Marketing, American Academy of Dermatology, USA; [c] Cronin Skin Cancer Center, Melbourne, FL, USA
* Corresponding author. Cronin Skin Cancer Center, 1399 S. Habor City Boulevard, Melbourne, FL 32901.
*E-mail address:* mcronin619@gmail.com

Dermatol Clin 44 (2026) 571–577
https://doi.org/10.1016/j.det.2026.06.002
0733-8635/26/

**Abbreviations**

| | |
|---|---|
| AAD | American Academy of Dermatology |
| COVID-19 | coronavirus disease 2019 |
| VMX | Virtual Meeting Experience |

In response, the AAD undertook a comprehensive, research-driven branding initiative aimed at aligning its identity, communications, and visual expression with its strategic priorities and member expectations. The goal of the AAD was not to simply have a "logo change" but to incorporate the fundamental practice of brand identity. This effort extended beyond visual redesign to include evaluation of member perceptions, development of a unified brand narrative, and implementation of a structured rollout and evaluation process. The following sections describe this process and illustrate how branding can function as a strategic, mission-driven framework within dermatology.

## THE AMERICAN ACADEMY OF DERMATOLOGY REBRANDING PROCESS

### *Foundational Research*

The rebranding process began with a structured assessment of existing brand equity and member perceptions to establish a data-driven foundation for subsequent decisions. This phase incorporated both qualitative and quantitative methodologies to capture a comprehensive view of stakeholder perspectives.

Qualitative research included 6 focus groups conducted with 33 members, providing detailed insight into how dermatologists experienced the organization and where they perceived opportunities for change. Quantitative analysis consisted of an online survey of 395 randomly selected members, enabling systematic evaluation of perceptions across domains such as education, advocacy, innovation, transparency, and organizational direction.[6]

Findings confirmed a strong baseline. Members expressed high levels of pride in the organization and consistently identified education as a central strength, with approximately 80% rating the AAD as effective or very effective in providing clinical education. Advocacy was similarly well regarded, with 85% of members recognizing the AAD as a leading voice for the specialty and 74% agreeing that it represents dermatology effectively in governmental settings. The organization was broadly described as relevant, practical, and welcoming, reinforcing its established role within the specialty.[6]

At the same time, the data identified areas of tension. Despite strong performance in core domains, the AAD was less frequently associated with attributes such as innovation, transparency, and responsiveness. Only a minority of members selected attributes such as "listens to me" or "modern and innovative," and approximately 40% perceived the organization as transparent, suggesting variability in how these characteristics were experienced.[6] Additionally, while the AAD was viewed as the voice of the specialty, fewer members felt that it represented individual dermatologists.

Taken together, these findings pointed to an opportunity to bridge established strengths and

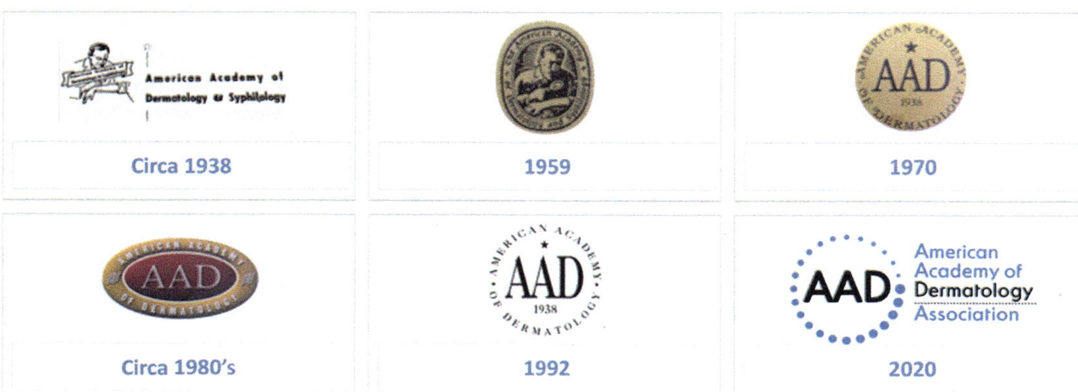


**Fig. 1.** Evolution of the American Academy of Dermatology (AAD) Logo and Visual Identity (1938–2020). The AAD logo has evolved over time in response to changes in professional practice, communication, and technology. Earlier designs reflected traditional institutional identity, while the 1992 logo remained in use for nearly 3 decades during a period of significant digital transformation. The 2020 redesign introduces a more contemporary visual system intended to reflect adaptability, connectivity, and the evolving expectations of members. This progression highlights that while the logo is a visible element of the brand, it reflects broader changes in organizational identity and context.

evolving expectations, providing the basis for defining a forward-looking direction.

### Defining the Future State

Building on these insights, the AAD articulated a future state aligned with its strategic planning efforts. This phase focused on defining how the organization intended to be perceived, rather than solely describing its current position. The future state positioned the AAD as a more adaptive and forward-looking organization, with increased emphasis on innovation, inclusivity, and engagement, while maintaining its established leadership in education and advocacy. This framing reflected an effort to align institutional identity with shifts in professional practice, communication, and member expectations.

By establishing this direction early in the process, the organization created a reference point against which subsequent decisions—including narrative development and design—could be evaluated. This step also set the stage for a more structured comparison between current perceptions and desired positioning.

### Gap Analysis

A formal gap analysis was conducted to compare current member perceptions with the defined future state, translating research findings into opportunities for realignment.

The analysis highlighted that existing strengths were not consistently reflected in how the organization was experienced or understood. Attributes such as innovation, transparency, and member responsiveness—identified as priorities in the future state—were variably perceived, indicating uneven visibility and communication across member groups. In addition, there was a distinction between the organization's role as a representative of the specialty and its perceived relevance to individual dermatologists. These findings suggested that the primary issue was not performance alone, but how that performance was interpreted and communicated.

### Development of the Brand Narrative

The brand narrative was developed as a response to the identified gaps, with the goal of creating a cohesive framework that could guide both strategic initiatives and communication. This narrative emphasized the concept of collective strength, positioning the AAD as an organization defined by the contributions and engagement of its members. Rather than introducing entirely new themes, the narrative reframed existing strengths—such as education and advocacy—while elevating areas requiring greater emphasis, including innovation and member engagement.[5]

In this context, the organization was presented not as a separate institutional entity but as a member-driven network, in which the collective expertise and participation of dermatologists shape its direction. This framing provided continuity with the organization's history while offering a clearer articulation of its evolving role. The narrative subsequently served as the foundation for visual identity development and implementation planning.

### Design Development and Logo Redesign

The design phase translated the brand narrative into a visual system intended to reflect both continuity and change. This process was iterative and informed by stakeholder input at multiple stages.

Initial development included 104 design concepts grouped into 11 directions, which were progressively refined to 61 designs and ultimately narrowed to a single direction following multiple rounds of evaluation. Stakeholder testing played a central role in this process, allowing the organization to assess how different design approaches were perceived and whether they aligned with the intended narrative. The final design reflects a balance between historical continuity and a more contemporary expression of the organization's identity. The retained blue color palette reinforces associations with trust and credibility that have long been linked to the AAD. Circular elements carry forward the visual language of the prior seal-like logo, preserving a sense of institutional heritage and recognition. At the same time, the introduction of a modern typographic system and a proprietary font reflects a shift toward a more current and adaptable identity.[6]

Additional design elements were used to convey the themes embedded in the brand narrative. A series of dots of varying sizes represents the membership itself—individual dermatologists contributing to a collective whole—while also suggesting diversity, movement, and ongoing evolution. The arrangement of these elements creates a sense of openness and forward motion, aligning with the organization's emphasis on innovation and engagement. The unified mark also integrates both the AAD and its advocacy arm within a single visual system, simplifying communication across platforms.

Rather than functioning as a purely esthetic update, the visual identity was developed as a direct extension of the brand narrative. In this way, the logo serves not only as a recognizable symbol but also as a condensed representation of the organization's values, priorities, and evolving role within dermatology.

## Implementation and Rollout

Implementation was structured to prioritize internal alignment before external introduction. Educational efforts were directed toward leadership, staff, and members to communicate the rationale behind the rebranding and the meaning of the new narrative. This included presentations at leadership meetings, departmental sessions to define "on-brand" initiatives, and early communication through Academy channels to familiarize members with the evolving brand framework.

External rollout was conducted through a coordinated, multiplatform communication strategy. Print and editorial platforms played a central role, including a series of articles in *Dermatology World* that introduced the branding initiative and sequentially outlined each narrative pillar—education, advocacy, member-centricity, and innovation. The official launch issue featured a redesigned cover, a gatefold promotional insert, and editorial content explaining the updated identity.

Digital platforms were used to extend reach and reinforce engagement. The AAD Web site (aad.org) served as a central hub for brand-related content, including videos, narrative explanations, and interactive features. Additional dissemination occurred through email campaigns, podcasts such as *Dialogues in Dermatology*, and social media channels, where member-facing initiatives—including ambassador-led campaigns and interactive "brand quizzes"—were used to encourage participation and familiarity with the new identity. These efforts were complemented by virtual programming, including presentations at the Virtual Meeting Experience (VMX), which provided an additional forum for introducing the brand in an educational context.[6]

Given the timing of the coronavirus disease 2019 (COVID-19) pandemic, the organization adopted a phased rollout strategy rather than a single large-scale launch. This approach emphasized gradual exposure, education, and reinforcement across multiple touchpoints. By integrating the new brand into existing communication channels and member interactions, the rollout allowed for adaptation to external conditions while maintaining continuity and engagement.

## Evaluation and Outcomes

Postimplementation evaluation focused on assessing awareness, perception, and alignment with the intended brand narrative. A follow-up survey of 814 members (12% response rate, ±3% margin of error) provided quantitative insight into these outcomes. Approximately half of respondents reported awareness of the rebranding, with higher recognition among younger members.[6] Across measured domains, agreement ratings increased relative to baseline, including perceptions of transparency, responsiveness, and innovation. For example, agreement that the AAD listens to members increased to approximately two-thirds of respondents, while perceptions of transparency improved but remained an area of variability.

Overall, approximately 71% of members reported satisfaction with how the organization was delivering on its brand promise. These findings suggest partial but measurable alignment between the intended narrative and member experience, while also indicating areas for continued refinement. This evaluation phase reinforced the understanding of branding as an ongoing process, providing a basis for continued adjustment and development.

## Operationalizing the Brand: Four Pillars of Transformation

The AAD operationalized its brand narrative through 4 core pillars—education, advocacy, member-centricity, and innovation—each representing both established strengths and areas identified for further development. These pillars functioned as organizing principles, translating research findings into specific initiatives and communication strategies that could be implemented across the organization.

### Education: from foundational strength to evolving standard

Education has long been a defining element of the AAD, serving as a primary driver of member engagement and professional identity. The rebranding process reframed education not only as a core function but also as an evolving commitment to deliver content that is practical, accessible, and aligned with contemporary practice. Existing educational platforms—including the Annual Meeting, *Journal of the American Academy of Dermatology*, and continuing medical education offerings—provided a strong foundation. Survey data indicated that approximately 80% of members rated the AAD as effective in delivering clinical education. Building on this foundation, the organization expanded its approach to include additional formats such as weekly digital learning tools (eg, Question of the Week), podcasts such as *Dialogues in Dermatology*, and immersive educational experiences through Innovation Academy.[7]

These initiatives reflected a shift toward delivering content that integrates into daily clinical practice while incorporating emerging topics such as digital health and evolving models of learning. In this context, education was positioned not only as a resource but also as a continuously developing component of professional growth.

### *Advocacy: from established voice to collective engagement*

Advocacy has historically been a central function of the AAD, supported by an established policy infrastructure and strong engagement with legislative and regulatory stakeholders. The rebranding process reframed advocacy to emphasize broader participation and visibility, extending beyond institutional representation. Quantitative data demonstrated that 85% of members viewed the AAD as the voice of the specialty, and 74% agreed that it effectively represents dermatology in government settings. At the same time, fewer members perceived the organization as representing individual dermatologists, highlighting an opportunity to expand engagement.

In response, advocacy efforts were positioned as a shared responsibility supported by organizational infrastructure. Initiatives included expansion of grassroots advocacy tools, increased visibility of campaigns such as SkinSerious, and broader use of digital platforms and social media to amplify messaging. The organization also continued to facilitate member participation through events such as the American Academy of Dermatology Association (AADA) Legislative Conference and online advocacy tools.[8]

This approach emphasized advocacy as a networked activity, in which institutional efforts are complemented by individual member participation, contributing to broader visibility within both policy and public domains.

### *Member-centricity: toward a listening and adaptive organization*

Member-centricity emerged as a key area for refinement, reflecting variability in how members experienced the organization's responsiveness and inclusivity. While the AAD was widely perceived as welcoming, survey findings indicated that a substantial proportion of members did not consistently perceive the organization as listening to their concerns. The rebranding process defined member-centricity as an ongoing effort to incorporate diverse perspectives while maintaining alignment around shared goals. This included expanding mechanisms for feedback collection, such as surveys, social media engagement, and direct member outreach, as well as reinforcing the role of dermatologist-led committees and advisory structures.[9]

The COVID-19 pandemic provided a context in which these principles could be operationalized. In response to rapidly changing clinical conditions, the AAD developed and disseminated guidance on telemedicine implementation, coding, practice management, and patient care considerations. Additional resources addressed questions related to treatment management, safety protocols, and practice reopening. These efforts reflected an approach focused on responsiveness and adaptability within a dynamic environment.

In this context, member-centricity functioned as an ongoing process rather than a fixed endpoint, emphasizing continuous alignment with member needs.

### *Innovation: facilitating change in practice and engagement*

Innovation was identified as an area where perception lagged behind existing capabilities. While members valued the organization's educational offerings, fewer associated the AAD with innovation or forward-looking approaches.

The rebranding process reframed innovation as the facilitation of new approaches to patient care, education, and member engagement. This included leveraging technology to enhance both clinical practice and organizational interaction.

Several initiatives reflected this shift. The development of the AAD VMX provided a fully digital educational platform with interactive sessions, live discussions, and on-demand content, attracting more than 4000 participants. This was followed by the introduction of the Academy's Innovation Academy, at the AAD's summer meeting. Web site redesign efforts focused on improving navigation and access to resources, incorporating features such as streamlined content organization and real-time communication tools. Additional innovations included expansion of virtual programming and adaptation of existing initiatives, such as Camp Discovery, into digital formats.[10]

These efforts positioned innovation as an enabling function, supporting adaptation to changing conditions while maintaining continuity in organizational offerings.

## Why Branding Matters in Dermatology

The AAD case situates branding not as a peripheral communication function, but as a mechanism through which organizational identity is clarified, interpreted, and sustained over time. In sociologic terms, branding can be understood as the outward expression of organizational identity—the set of attributes that are central, distinctive, and enduring—and as a tool for maintaining institutional legitimacy within a broader professional and public context.[6,11] Within dermatology, where professional identity is shaped across clinical, academic, and public-facing domains, branding provides a structured way to align how the specialty understands itself with how it is perceived by others.

The findings from the AAD rebranding process suggest that misalignment does not necessarily arise from absence of performance, but from variability in how that performance is interpreted. This reflects the concept of sensemaking, in which stakeholders construct meaning based on available signals and experiences. In this context, branding functions as a coordinating framework, helping to reduce ambiguity by making organizational priorities more visible and coherent.[12] The emphasis on narrative development and consistent messaging across platforms can be viewed as an effort to stabilize interpretation across a diverse membership.

Branding also contributes to internal alignment, particularly in organizations characterized by heterogeneous stakeholders.[13] Dermatology includes a range of practice settings, subspecialties, and career stages, each associated with different expectations of professional organizations. The AAD's focus on member-centricity and collective identity reflects an attempt to balance these differences while maintaining a shared direction. In this way, branding operates as a mechanism for organizing diversity rather than eliminating it, allowing variation to coexist within a unified framework.[6]

At the same time, branding has implications beyond the organization itself. It shapes how dermatology is positioned within the broader health care system and how its value is communicated to policymakers, other specialties, and the public.[2,14–19] The emphasis on advocacy as a "collective voice" highlights the role of branding in amplifying professional representation, particularly in environments where visibility and recognition influence policy and resource allocation. Similarly, the focus on innovation reflects the need to align the specialty with evolving expectations around technology, access, and care delivery.

These dynamics extend to the level of clinical practice. Dermatology practices increasingly operate in environments where patient perception is influenced by digital platforms, online reviews, and social media presence.[2,15–19] In this setting, branding contributes to how expertise is interpreted, how trust is established, and how continuity is maintained across patient interactions.[20–23] The principles observed in the AAD rebranding case—consistency, clarity of purpose, and alignment between identity and experience—are therefore applicable at both organizational and practice levels.[24–27]

## LIMITATION

Several limitations should be considered when interpreting the findings from the AAD rebranding evaluation. First, the follow-up member survey had a response rate of 12%,[6] which may have introduced response bias, as respondents may not have been fully representative of the broader AAD membership. Individuals with greater engagement with the organization may have been more likely to participate, resulting in potential overrepresentation of their perspectives. Second, although descriptive differences were observed between baseline and follow-up survey measures, formal statistical testing was not performed for prerebranding and postrebranding comparisons. Thus, the significance and magnitude of the observed changes cannot be definitively established. Third, the evaluation lacked a control condition or comparison group, limiting the ability to attribute observed changes solely to the rebranding initiative. External factors, including secular trends, evolving member expectations, and broader societal influences such as the COVID-19 pandemic and its downstream effects on professional organizations and communication practices, may also have contributed to shifts in member perceptions.

## SUMMARY

The AAD rebranding initiative provides an example of branding as a structured, research-informed process that integrates organizational identity with evolving expectations. By linking member perceptions to narrative development, design, and implementation, the process illustrates how branding can be used to coordinate internal priorities and external representation without disrupting established strengths.

More broadly, branding in dermatology may be viewed as an ongoing process of alignment rather than a discrete intervention. As the specialty continues to evolve in response to changes in care delivery, communication, and professional expectations, the ability to articulate a coherent and adaptable identity remains central to maintaining relevance.

## CLINICS CARE POINTS

- With the rebranding effort it was found that education and advocacy with existing strengths to reframe a pitfall to this was that other areas such as innovation and member engagmenet were in need of elevation.
- Having less member engagment would weaken any future branding efforts.

## FUNDING

Funding for study was given by American Academy of Dermatology.

## DISCLOSURE

Ms M. Hall serves within the Growth, Brand & Partnerships division of the American Academy of Dermatology (AAD) Communication & Marketing department, which was involved in the implementation of the AAD rebranding initiative described in this article. This affiliation is disclosed in the interest of transparency and may represent an institutional perspective relevant to the subject matter. The remaining authors report no conflicts of interest.

## REFERENCES

1. Elrod JK, Fortenberry JL Jr. Driving brand equity in health services organizations: the need for an expanded view of branding. BMC Health Serv Res 2018;18(Suppl 3):924.
2. Berry LL, Bendapudi N. Clueing in customers. Harv Bus Rev 2003;81(2):100–26.
3. Brennan MD, Monson V. Professionalism: good for patients and health care organizations. Mayo Clin Proc 2014;89(5):644–52.
4. Platt J, Goold SD. Betraying, earning, or justifying trust in health organizations. Hastings Cent Rep 2023;53(Suppl 2):S53–9.
5. Burgdorf WH, Bickers DR. Dermatologic relationships between the United States and german-speaking countries. Part I--before 1933. JAMA Dermatol 2013;149(8):966–9.
6. American Academy of Dermatology. Why branding matters. Seattle (WA): Innovation Academy; 2024.
7. Hall MT. Education: from go-to to gold standard. Schaumburg (IL): Dermatol World; 2020. p. 50–1.
8. Hall MT. Advocacy: from voice to collective impact. Schaumburg (IL): Dermatol World; 2020. p. 56–8.
9. Hall MT. Member-centricity: becoming a listening organization. Dermatol World 2020;56–8.
10. Hall MT. Innovation: advancing dermatology through new approaches. Dermatol World 2020;58–60.
11. Salvatore D, Numerato D, Fattore G. Physicians' professional autonomy and their organizational identification with their hospital. BMC Health Serv Res 2018;18(1):775.
12. Kelm RC, Ibrahim O. Modernizing marketing strategies for social media and millennials in dermatology. Clin Dermatol 2023;41(2):246–52.
13. Shanafelt TD, Wang H, Leonard M, et al. Assessment of the association of leadership behaviors of supervising physicians with personal-organizational values alignment among staff physicians. JAMA Netw Open 2021;4(2):e2035622.
14. Cruess RL, Cruess SR. Professionalism, communities of practice, and medicine's social contract. J Am Board Fam Med 2020;33(Suppl):S50–6.
15. Forgie EME, Lai H, Cao B, et al. Social media and the transformation of the physician-patient relationship: viewpoint. J Med Internet Res 2021;23(12):e25230.
16. Górska-Warsewicz H. Consumer or patient determinants of hospital brand equity—A systematic literature review. Int J Environ Res Publ Health 2022;19(15):9026.
17. Elrod JK, Fortenberry JL. Driving brand equity in health services organizations: the need for an expanded view of branding. BMC Health Serv Res 2018;18(Suppl 3):924.
18. Corbin CL, Kelley SW, Schwartz RW. Concepts in service marketing for healthcare professionals. Am J Surg 2001;181(1):1–7.
19. Branzetti J, Gisondi MA, Hopson LR, et al. Physician, know thyself: applying brand management principles to professional identity in academic medicine. Med Educ 2025;59(7):694–703.
20. Elrod JK, Fortenberry JL. Response hierarchy models and their application in health and medicine: understanding the hierarchy of effects. BMC Health Serv Res 2020;20(Suppl 1):824.
21. Kream EJ, Jerdan K. Digital brand building and online reputation management in dermatology. Clin Dermatol 2023;41(2):240–5.
22. Murphy EC, Nelson K, Friedman AJ. The influence of dermatologists' use of social media on attracting patients. J Drugs Dermatol JDD 2020;19(5):532–8.
23. Smith RJ, Lipoff JB. Evaluation of dermatology practice online reviews: lessons from qualitative analysis. JAMA Dermatol 2016;152(2):153–7.
24. Keller KL. Conceptualizing, measuring, and managing customer-based brand equity. J Market 1993;57(1):1–22.
25. Keller KL. Strategic brand management: building, measuring, and managing brand equity. 5th edition. London, UK: Pearson; 2019.
26. Aaker DA. Managing brand equity: capitalizing on the value of a brand name. New York City (NY): Free Press; 1991.
27. Aaker DA. Building strong brands. New York City (NY): Free Press; 1996.

# Being a Social Media Ambassador

Brittani Remé, DO, MS, Oyetewa Asempa, MD, FAAD*

**KEYWORDS**

• Social media • Dermatology education • Advocacy • Instagram • TikTok • YouTube • Facebook • X

**KEY POINTS**

- Social media has become a primary source of information for dermatology conditions for patients.
- Dermatologists play a crucial role as trusted educators on social media.
- Engaging on social media can provide the public access to evidence-based skin care, improve health literacy, and combat misinformation.
- Serving as a social media ambassador for the specialty requires employing platform-specific strategies and transparency while adhering to professional and ethical standards.

## BACKGROUND

To understand the modern role of the dermatologist as a social media ambassador, we must first appreciate how recently and how profoundly social media has reshaped communication. The public Internet became mainstream in the early 1990s. Social media platforms emerged in the late 1990s and early 2000s and solidified into cultural and economic institutions by approximately 2005. What began as a tool for college students to connect with peers has evolved into a global infrastructure for information exchange, opinion formation, marketing, and commerce.

As of 2025, the global population is approximately 8.3 billion.[1] An estimated 6 billion individuals use the Internet, and 5.66 billion maintain active social media identities.[2] This represents nearly 70% of humanity. Social media is now the largest communication network in history and one of the most powerful tools ever created for building scalable human connection.

For dermatologists, this digital ecosystem presents significant professional opportunity. Social media can serve as a platform for

- Professional networking with physicians and allied providers across institutions
- Research collaboration and exchange of practice innovation
- Responsible brand partnerships
- Practice growth through expanded visibility
- Public education, advocacy, and dissemination of evidence-based information

At the same time, social media exists within a broader shift in how patients seek and interpret health information. Increasingly, patients turn to digital platforms for health information before seeking professional care. The 2024 State of Consumer Health survey by Healthline found that among 4012 adults in the United States, fewer than half, 37%, identified a doctor or health care professional as their preferred source of health information.[3] Over the previous 12 months, 52% reported trying wellness tactics after learning about them on social media. The survey also noted that some patients are missing routine screenings while simultaneously experimenting with health trends encountered online.

Department of Dermatology, Baylor College of Medicine, 1977 Butler Boulevard, E6.200, Houston, TX 77030, USA
* Corresponding author.
*E-mail address:* oyetewaoyerinde@gmail.com

Dermatol Clin 44 (2026) 579–587
https://doi.org/10.1016/j.det.2026.05.003

**Abbreviations**

| | |
|---|---|
| AI | artificial intelligence |
| FAAD | Fellow of the American Academy of Dermatology |

Patients are drawn to social media for understandable reasons.[4] They seek

- Empowerment through easily accessible knowledge
- Digestible and relatable medical content
- Practical guidance on navigating chronic conditions
- Validation of their lived experiences
- Community and belonging

Simultaneously, patients consistently reject:

- Judgmental tone
- Invalidation of their concerns
- Talking down about other professionals

While social media offers access and relatability, it also accelerates the spread of misinformation. A 2023 study evaluating the 100 most viewed YouTube videos related to emergency general surgical procedures, including appendectomy and cholecystectomy, revealed substantial deficiencies in quality.[5] Using validated instruments, investigators found that 49% of videos provided no meaningful patient education, and 35% contained misinformation. Content produced by physicians and health care systems contained significantly less misinformation than content produced by patients or wellness groups.

Dermatology faces similar challenges. Viral TikTok challenges such as the "sunburn challenge" of 2022 have normalized behaviors that directly contradict established dermatologic science and skin cancer prevention principles.[6]

The implications for our specialty are clear. Social media is now one of the primary spaces in which patients form beliefs about their skin, hair, and nail health. If dermatologists are absent from these conversations, others will define the narrative.[7] Meeting patients where they already are provides an opportunity to educate, empower, and guide with evidence-based information. Building credibility and long term trust will allow us to shape public understanding of dermatologic expertise.

This article examines social media as a central tool for connection, credibility, and influence within leadership, branding, and the business of dermatology, while also providing a detailed, practical guide to establishing a presence on social media, growing a following, and building a professional brand.

## THE EXPANDING ROLE OF SOCIAL MEDIA IN DERMATOLOGY

The expanding role of social media use within dermatology reflects a structural shift in how patients access information, evaluate expertise, and select clinicians.[7] As dermatology sits at the intersection of medical disease, preventive medicine, procedural care, and esthetics, the implications and consequences of widespread misinformation are substantial. For this reason, academic dermatologists, private practice physicians, researchers, residency programs and directors, and subspecialty experts alike have a role to play in representing the specialty online.

### *Why Dermatologists Should Engage*

Patients are already present in digital spaces seeking guidance. If dermatologists do not actively participate, the information landscape will be defined by nonphysician voices, commercial interests, or misinformation. At both individual and collective levels, presence reinforces dermatology's identity as the true domain experts in cutaneous medicine.

Active participation enables dermatologists to[8]

- Position themselves and the specialty as the authoritative source for skin, hair, and nail health
- Extend patient education beyond the clinical encounter
- Enhance institutional, academic, and practice visibility
- Support recruitment, research dissemination, and professional advancement

### *Combatting Misinformation on Social Media*

The digital ecosystem allows individuals without formal training to present themselves as authorities. Differentiation is therefore essential. Dermatologists must clearly signal credentials, training, and scope of expertise while delivering evidence-based content that is accessible and clinically accurate.

Effective differentiation includes explicit identification as a board-certified dermatologist and Fellow of the American Academy of Dermatology (FAAD) and visible alignment with evidence-based medicine. When misinformation or unsafe trends emerge, responses should focus on explaining the absence of scientific support, outlining potential risks, and referencing reputable sources.[9]

### *Establishing Credibility on Social Media as a Dermatologist*

Patient privacy must remain paramount, with written consent obtained prior to sharing any images or stories and strict adherence to institutional and legal standards.

Long-term credibility also depends on maintaining an appropriate balance between educational and promotional content, preserving professionalism, and engaging thoughtfully with audiences. Content that disparages other professionals or patients undermines both individual and specialty credibility. Responsive, measured engagement with questions and comments can strengthen trust while maintaining appropriate boundaries.

## FOUNDATIONS OF CONTENT CREATION

The foundations of content creation require clarity of purpose, alignment of audience and platform, and disciplined execution (**Fig. 1**). Without these elements, even clinically accurate content may fail to resonate with the public.

### *Determining Your Purpose*

Clarity of purpose shapes tone, content type, frequency, and long-term strategy.

Common motivations include

- Building a professional brand to support product development or consulting
- Marketing a clinical practice
- Growing a community around a shared condition or interest
- Providing public education without commercial goals
- Offering educational content that is engaging or entertaining

A dermatologist whose goal is to market a procedural practice will create different content than one focused on academic thought leadership or patient education. Ambiguity at this stage often results in inconsistent messaging and limited growth.

### *Selecting a Niche*

A defined niche clarifies identity and differentiates one's content in an increasingly saturated space. The niche should align with clinical expertise, authentic interest, and audience demand. Potential niches are endless, but include

- Hair loss and scalp disorders
- Complex medical dermatology
- Cosmetic dermatology
- Pediatric dermatology
- Skin of color
- Pregnancy-related skin concerns

### *Selecting a Target Audience*

Content is most effective when tailored to a clearly defined audience. Dermatologists should consider age, gender, life stage, cultural background, and health concerns. For example, content designed for pregnant or expecting mothers will differ in tone and emphasis from content targeting adolescents with acne or more mature adults concerned about aging.

### *Selecting a Platform*

Platform selection should align with both content style and target audience behavior. Each platform privileges distinct formats and user expectations.[10] Moreover, content trends evolve rapidly, often faster than traditional publishing cycles. Dermatologists should remain attentive to real-time shifts in platform algorithms and audience preferences (**Table 1**).

Selecting 1 primary platform initially allows focused effort. Platform-specific considerations include[11]

- Facebook, where videos and longer written posts remain relevant
- Instagram, which prioritizes short-form video through reels and educational carousels
- YouTube, which favors long-form educational videos and vlogs
- TikTok, where video predominates, though still images are gaining traction
- X (Twitter), which emphasizes concise commentary, academic discourse, and clinical updates

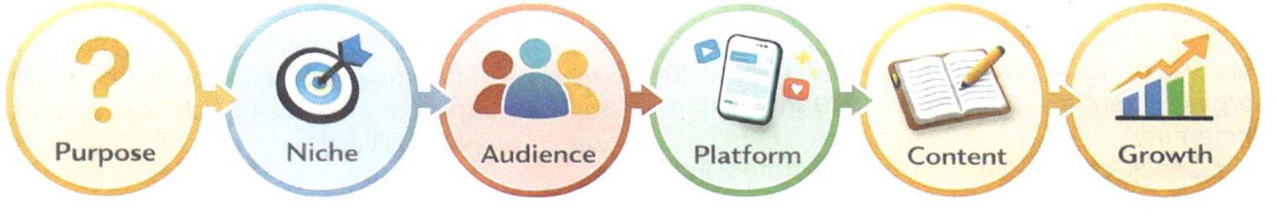


**Fig. 1.** Steps to building a strong foundation for content creation: (1) determining your purpose, (2) selecting a niche, (3) selecting a target audience, (4) selecting a platform, (5) content planning, and (6) optimizing for growth.

**Table 1**
**Social media platform specific applications in dermatology**

| Platform | Primary Audience | Dermatology-related Content |
|---|---|---|
| Facebook | Ages 65 y and older are the platform's demographic, 84% of US Millennials are active users of the social media platform | Patient support pages<br>Medical journals sharing content<br>Professional society and event promotion<br>Residency information pages |
| Instagram | 60% of users are aged 18–34 y, young adults and Millennials | Before-and-after images<br>Videos of disease info and procedures<br>Product promotion<br>Residency information |
| YouTube | Percentage of people on YouTube is evenly spread across the various age groups | Product promotion<br>Long-form videos of dermatologic information and procedures<br>Educational video libraries |
| TikTok | Largest user group is age 10–19 y (gen Z), although the app is widely used by many age groups | Myth-busting of viral trends<br>Product promotion<br>Photos/videos of dermatologic information and procedures |
| X (Twitter) | 25–34 y olds: 38.5% of users, and 70.4% of Twitter's user base identifies as male individuals, while only 29.6% are female individuals | Medical journals sharing content<br>Dermatology topic discussions<br>Public health messaging |
| LinkedIn | Professionals aged 25–49 y, including physicians, researchers, administrators, and industry leaders | Thought leadership articles<br>Research dissemination and academic achievements<br>Professional announcements and career milestones |

- LinkedIn, which emphasizes professional articles and thought leadership

### *Practical Tips for Planning and Social Media Management*

Strategic planning can occur at multiple time horizons:

*Quarterly planning* allows dermatologists to brainstorm themes relevant to their niche and audience. Awareness months and health observances provide timely anchors for educational content.

*Monthly planning* involves mapping out specific posts, aligning them with awareness campaigns and clinical priorities. Weekly batching of content production is efficient. Preparing talking points, attire, and visual props in advance enables filming of multiple short videos in a single session.

*Daily engagement* includes monitoring comments, responding thoughtfully, and observing emerging trends that may warrant timely commentary.

Awareness campaigns can be integrated into content calendars. Examples include

- January—Thyroid Awareness Month
- February—American Heart Month and World Cancer Day on February 4
- March—National Doctor's Day on March 30
- April—Rosacea Awareness Month
- May—Skin Cancer Awareness Month, Melanoma Monday on the first Monday, and Don't Fry Day on the last Friday
- June—Acne Awareness Month, Vitiligo Awareness Month, and World Vitiligo Day on June 25
- August—Hair Loss Awareness Month and Psoriasis Awareness Month
- September—Healthy Aging Month
- October—Eczema Awareness Month and World Psoriasis Day on October 29
- November—National Healthy Skin Month

Social media management platforms such as Zoho Social, Buffer, Hootsuite, Sprout Social, and Social Pilot can streamline scheduling, cross posting, and analytics tracking. Utilizing such tools enhances efficiency and sustainability, particularly for dermatologists balancing clinical and academic responsibilities.

## HOW TO CREATE MEANINGFUL CONTENT

Dermatologists occupy a uniquely visual specialty, which provides both opportunity and responsibility in digital communication. Meaningful content is educational, ethically sound, professionally presented, and strategically constructed to foster trust and engagement.

### *Content Types*

Frequently asked questions in the clinic often serve as a rich source of social media content ideas. Transforming repetitive in-clinic explanations into short, accessible educational posts enhances efficiency and broadens impact.[12] Common content types include

- Short-form videos explaining common conditions, procedures, or myths
- Long-form educational videos exploring complex concepts or tutorials
- Before and after images that establish credibility and set realistic expectations
- Infographics and carousel posts presenting concise, shareable facts
- Product reviews grounded in evidence and clinical experience
- Myth busting posts addressing viral trends
- Question and answer videos based on frequently asked clinical questions
- Day in the life content that humanizes the physician
- Live sessions featuring interviews with experts or real-time audience interaction
- Stories that build rapport through behind-the-scenes insights

To build rapport and trust, dermatologists should

- Use accessible language and minimize unnecessary jargon
- Communicate with compassion and clarity
- Post consistently, ideally a minimum of 2 to 3 times weekly for short-form content (such as on Instagram and TikTok, or YouTube Shorts) and weekly for long-form content (such as full-length YouTube videos)
- When appropriate, share success stories or testimonials with proper consent

### *Equipment*

High-quality content does not require immediate investment in professional equipment. Early stage creators can effectively use a smartphone, a simple tripod, and natural light. Filming directly in front of a window with a neutral background provides sufficient illumination and professionalism. Waiting for perfect equipment often delays action.

Filming should occur in a quiet, well-lit environment. A tripod stabilizes the device and improves visual quality. As content production becomes more sophisticated, additional tools may be incorporated, including a wireless microphone for improved audio clarity and a ring light to supplement lighting when natural light is insufficient (**Fig. 2**).

For advanced content creation, dermatologists may invest in a professional camera, larger lighting systems, backdrops, or a dedicated recording space within the home or office to ensure consistent visual standards.

### *Editing Tools*

Many platforms offer in app editing tools such as Instagram Edits and TikTok's native editor. These tools are sufficient for basic trimming, captions, and formatting.

Third-party applications expand capabilities. Canva, Captions, CapCut, iMovie, Animoto, and Lightroom offer options for video editing, graphic design, subtitles, and color correction. Numerous free or low-cost applications exist that streamline workflow and improve production quality without requiring extensive technical expertise.

### *Artificial Intelligence and Content Creation*

Artificial intelligence (AI) tools are now increasingly integrated into the content creation process. Platforms such as ChatGPT, Claude, Gemini, and Microsoft Copilot can assist with generating topic ideas, drafting scripts, outlining educational posts, summarizing research, and refining language for clarity and accessibility.[13] Design-oriented AI tools

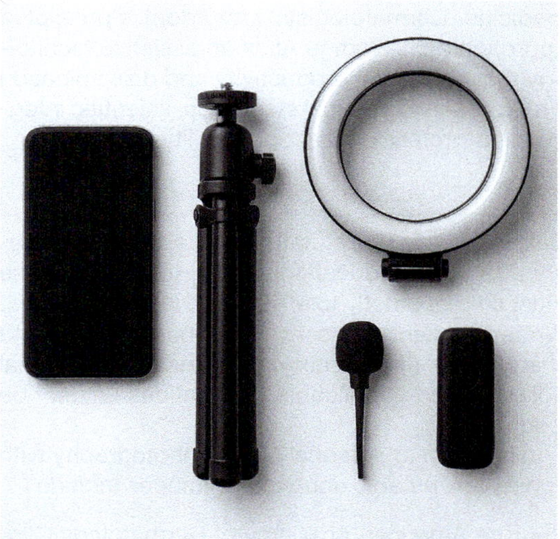

**Fig. 2.** Basic equipment for content creation, including cell phone, tripod, ring light, and wireless microphone.

such as Canva Magic Design, Adobe Firefly, and Midjourney can support infographic development and visual concept generation. For literature identification and citation support, tools such as OpenEvidence, Consensus, Semantic Scholar, and Elicit can help surface peer-reviewed studies and synthesize research findings relevant to specific claims.

When used appropriately, these tools can enhance efficiency and expand creative capacity.[14] They may assist dermatologists in translating complex pathophysiology into patient-friendly explanations, structuring content series, generating frequently asked question scripts, or identifying emerging topics in the literature.

However, AI-generated output must never substitute for clinical expertise or scholarly rigor.[14] Dermatologists remain fully responsible for the accuracy, safety, and appropriateness of any content disseminated under their name. All AI-assisted scripts, graphics, and summaries require careful review to ensure alignment with current guidelines, appropriate nuance in areas of controversy, and accurate representation of evidence. Particular scrutiny should be applied to therapeutic recommendations, safety data, and emerging research.

Transparency is equally important. When AI tools play a substantive role in content development, especially in educational materials or research summaries, disclosure may be appropriate depending on context, audience, and institutional policy. Transparency supports trust and aligns with evolving norms in academic and professional communication.

AI will undoubtedly assume a larger role in digital medicine. Dermatologists who adopt a principled approach can leverage AI as an assistive technology that enhances productivity and dissemination while preserving ethical standards, scientific integrity, and professional accountability.

### Adding Clinical Photos into Content

Dermatology's visual nature makes clinical imagery a powerful educational tool. However, its use must adhere strictly to ethical and legal standards. Written patient consent is mandatory prior to sharing identifiable clinical images. Institutional policies and applicable regulations must be followed.

In addition to personal clinical photography with consent, reputable sources for images include

- The American Academy of Dermatology Clinical Image Collection
- DermNet NZ, ensuring watermark visibility per their current guidelines
- Peer-reviewed journals such as *Journal of the American Academy of Dermatology* and *Journal of the American Medical Association Dermatology* with appropriate citation
- VisualDx, where written permission may be requested through the Image Collection Manager

### Tips for Growth

Growth is a function of both content quality and strategic behavior. Several principles consistently influence audience expansion.[15]

- Engagement matters. Responding to comments and fostering dialog strengthens community and signals credibility to platform algorithms.
- Consistency is more important than sporadic volume. Regular posting establishes audience expectations and reinforces expertise.
- Brevity enhances retention. Content under 1 minute often performs best for educational videos.
- Professional networking supports growth. Following and engaging with colleagues can foster collaboration and expand reach.
- Participation in relevant trends, when aligned with professional standards, increases discoverability.
- Authenticity sustains trust. Audiences respond to genuine communication more than formulaic branding.
- Finally, data analysis is indispensable. Professional or creator accounts provide insights into optimal posting times, audience demographics, and engagement metrics. Monitoring analytics enables refinement of strategy and identification of monetization tools where appropriate.

## CASE STUDY

The following case study illustrates how strategic alignment of purpose, platform, niche, and audience can translate into meaningful digital impact within dermatology. It reflects the experience of a board-certified dermatologist specializing in hair loss and scalp disorders who leveraged social media as both an educational and leadership tool.

### Professional Profile

The physician is a dermatologist with focused expertise in hair loss and scalp disorders. The primary platform selected was Instagram. The niche was clearly defined as hair and scalp disorders, with a particular emphasis on women of color. The target audience consisted of women of color experiencing hair loss, a population in whom certain scarring alopecias are prevalent yet frequently underdiagnosed.

This specificity allowed for alignment among clinical expertise, lived patient experience, and digital messaging.

### *Clarifying Purpose*

The motivation for engagement was 2 fold: public education and brand and community building.

Educational objectives included

- Providing accessible patient information
- Combating misinformation regarding hair growth, styling practices, and treatment options
- Increasing awareness of underdiagnosed hair disorders in a demographic historically marginalized in research and representation.

Community and brand objectives included

- Establishing expertise in skin of color and hair disorders
- Creating a psychologically safe space for patients experiencing hair loss
- Expanding opportunities for public speaking and professional leadership

The integration of these goals shaped tone, topic selection, and long-term strategy. Education and advocacy were prioritized over purely promotional content.

### *Content Brainstorming and Strategy*

By translating frequently asked questions into concise, shareable posts, the content remained clinically relevant and audience-centered. Content development was rooted in common patient questions encountered in clinic, such as

- Why is my hair falling out?
- What is the best way to regrow hair?
- Are certain hairstyles contributing to my hair loss?

Because hair loss is deeply personal and emotionally charged, compassion informed all messaging. Tone was deliberate, validating patient experiences while providing evidence-based guidance. Content strategies included

- Before and after photographs demonstrating treatment progress and setting realistic expectations
- Video tutorials outlining best practices for hair care at home
- Infographics explaining common causes of hair loss
- Myth busting posts addressing influencer driven misinformation

### *Impact and Lessons*

This case study demonstrates that meaningful digital engagement is not accidental. It requires clear identification of a clinical niche, defined audience alignment, explicit articulation of educational and leadership goals, compassionate, evidence-based communication, and strategic use of both short-form and long-form platforms.

For dermatologists seeking to serve as social media ambassadors, this case underscores a central principle: precision of purpose, authenticity of voice, and disciplined execution can transform social media from a promotional tool into a platform for education, leadership, and measurable professional growth.

## ETHICAL CONSIDERATIONS AND PROFESSIONAL STANDARDS

As dermatologists expand their presence in digital spaces, ethical obligations remain constant, though the scale and permanence of social media amplify both opportunity and risk. Professionalism online must be intentional. The credibility of the individual physician and the integrity of the specialty depend on disciplined adherence to ethical standards.[16]

First, dermatologists must clearly distinguish between general education and individualized medical advice. Public posts should include language clarifying that content is for informational purposes only and does not replace a formal clinical evaluation. Refraining from offering patient-specific guidance in comments or direct messages protects both the physician and the public, while reinforcing appropriate clinical boundaries.

Confidentiality remains paramount. Written and specific social media consent must be obtained before posting identifiable patient photographs, before and after images, or testimonials. Even deidentified cases require caution to prevent inadvertent disclosure. Compliance with institutional policies and applicable privacy regulations is essential.

Dermatologists affiliated with academic centers or health systems should consult legal or media officers before posting content that could be interpreted as representing the institution. Transparency regarding potential conflicts of interest, including brand partnerships or advisory roles, is equally critical. Clear disclosure preserves trust and aligns with professional and regulatory expectations.

Professional conduct online should reflect the same standards upheld in clinic. Content should be consistent with what one would present in front of a patient or colleague. Public disparagement of other professionals, argumentative exchanges with followers, or emotionally reactive posts undermine credibility and erode trust. Engagement must remain respectful and measured, even when correcting misinformation.

Ethical discipline ensures that social media engagement strengthens, rather than compromises, the authority of dermatologists as experts in skin, hair, and nail health.

## SUMMARY

Social media has fundamentally reshaped how patients access information and evaluate expertise. For dermatologists, digital engagement is no longer optional. It is intertwined with leadership, branding, education, and the long-term positioning of the specialty. This article has outlined the responsibility to meet patients where they are with evidence-based, compassionate communication while countering misinformation and reinforcing dermatologists as the true experts in skin, hair, and nail health.

Effective engagement requires clarity of purpose, strategic platform use, thoughtful content creation, ethical discipline, and professionalism consistent with clinical practice. When approached intentionally, social media becomes more than a marketing tool. It becomes a vehicle for education, advocacy, community building, and the sustained elevation of dermatology.

## CLINICS CARE POINTS

- Clearly state that your content is educational and not individualized medical advice. Do not provide patient-specific recommendations in comments or direct messages.
- Obtain written, explicit social media consent before posting any patient photos, testimonials, or before and after images.
- Identify yourself consistently as a board-certified dermatologist and include FAAD in your bio and, when appropriate, in posts.
- Anchor claims in evidence. Cite reputable sources when correcting misinformation or discussing treatments.
- Define a specific niche and target audience to strengthen authority and clarity of messaging.
- Post consistently, prioritizing clarity and brevity.
- Maintain professionalism at all times. Do not argue with followers or disparage other professionals.
- Review all AI-assisted content carefully for scientific accuracy before posting.

## DECLARATION OF ARTIFICIAL INTELLIGENCE AND ARTIFICIAL INTELLIGENCE-ASSISTED TECHNOLOGIES IN THE WRITING PROCESS

During the preparation of this article, the authors used ChatGPT in order to edit for wording structure. After using this tool/service, the authors reviewed and edited the content as needed and take full responsibility for the content of the publication.

## DISCLOSURE

None.

## REFERENCES

1. United Nations Department of Economic and Social Affairs, population division. World population prospects: the 2019 revision population database. Version 2019; released January 2026. United Nations. Available at: https://population.un.org/wpp/. Accessed February 15, 2026.
2. International Telecommunication Union. Almost three-quarters of the population are online. ITU DataHub/Statistics (Facts and figures 2025—Internet use). 2025. Available at: https://www.itu.int/itu-d/reports/statistics/2025/10/15/ff25-internet-use/. Accessed February 15, 2026.
3. Healthline media. State of consumer health. Healthline. 2024. Available at: https://www.healthline.com/health/consumer-health-survey. Accessed February 15, 2026.
4. Gantenbein L, Navarini AA, Maul LV, et al. Internet and social media use in dermatology patients: search behavior and impact on patient-physician relationship. Dermatol Ther 2020;33(6):e14098.
5. Roberts B, Kobritz M, Nofi C, et al. Social media, misinformation, and online patient education in emergency general surgical procedures. J Surg Res 2023;287:16–23.
6. TikTok to ban videos that encourage sunburn and tanning after alarm from medical experts. The Guardian. 2022. Available at: https://www.theguardian.com/technology/2022/dec/01/tiktok-to-ban-videos-that-encourage-sunburn-and-tanning-after-alarm-from-medical-experts. Accessed February 15, 2026.
7. Lammer M, Wanner M, Bellmann P, et al. Integrating social media into modern dermatology - a cross-sectional study. J Dtsch Dermatol Ges 2025. https://doi.org/10.1111/ddg.15911.
8. Wojtara MS. Use of social media for patient education in dermatology: narrative review. JMIR Dermatol 2023;6:e42609.
9. Vraga EK, Bode L. Correction as a solution for health misinformation on social media. Am J Publ Health 2020;110(S3):S278–80.

10. Dinh T. Biggest social media platforms by users 2025. Statista. 2025. Available at: https://www.statista.com/statistics/272014/global-social-networks-ranked-by-number-of-users/. Accessed January 20, 2026.
11. Cooper BR, Concilla A, Albrecht JM, et al. Social media as a medium for dermatologic education. Curr Dermatol Rep 2022;11(2):103–9.
12. Kite J, Chan L, MacKay K, et al. A model of social media effects in public health communication campaigns: systematic review. J Med Internet Res 2023;25:e46345.
13. Boscardin CK, Gin B, Golde PB, et al. ChatGPT and generative artificial intelligence for medical education: potential impact and opportunity. Acad Med 2024;99(1):22–7.
14. Izquierdo-Condoy JS, Arias-Intriago M, Tello-De-la-Torre A, et al. Generative artificial intelligence in medical education: enhancing critical thinking or undermining cognitive autonomy? J Med Internet Res 2025;27:e76340.
15. Kream EJ, Jerdan K. Digital brand building and online reputation management in dermatology. Clin Dermatol 2023;41(2):240–5.
16. American Academy of Dermatology. Position statement on medical professionalism in the use of social media. American Academy of Dermatology. Approved April 28, 2018. Amended May 3, 2025. 2025. Available at: https://server.aad.org/forms/policies/Uploads/PS/PS-MedicalProfessionalismintheUseofSocialMedia.pdf. Accessed January 20, 2026.

# Pearls and Pitfalls of Social Media in Dermatology

Lorena Oliveira Fonseca, MD[a,b,*], Katherine Plampton, MD[b], Ronda Farah, MD FAAD[a,b]

**KEYWORDS**

- Social media • Dermatology • Digital professionalism • Physician branding
- Online patient education • Marketing in medicine

**KEY POINTS**

- Social media is a core component of dermatologic communication and professionalism.
- Clear purpose, consistent branding, and high-quality content improve credibility and audience trust.
- Ethical standards, Health Insurance Portability and Accountability Act, consent, and avoidance of personalized medical advice must guide all online activity.
- Strategic workflows and realistic posting habits support sustainability and reduce digital burnout.
- Awareness of Food and Drug Administration and medical board rules is essential to avoid regulatory and medicolegal risk.

## INTRODUCTION

Social media has quickly become one of the most powerful communication tools in modern medicine. Dermatology is a field that benefits greatly from the use of digital platforms because of its reliance on visual presentation, current trends, and direct interaction with patients Instagram, TikTok, YouTube, Threads, X, and new apps significant influence patient expectations before they visit the clinic. These platforms also serve as open forums where skin care myths spread rapidly, esthetic trends shift overnight, and commercial messages compete directly with medical knowledge.[1–3]

Much of the dermatology content online comes from non-physician influencers, estheticians, cosmetic practitioners, and industry partners. Board-certified dermatologists, despite having the most appropriate qualifications to inform the public, represent only a small portion of these voices.[3] This imbalance raises the risk of misinformation and highlights the need for dermatologists to maintain a thoughtful, ethical, and trustworthy presence online.[4,5]

This article outlines practical tips and common mistakes to assist dermatologists in creating sustainable, professional, and reliable digital identities. It emphasizes clear strategy, realistic workflow, ethical communication, and long-term engagement instead of high-volume posting or trend chasing.

## DISCUSSION

### *Pearl 1: Define Your Purpose before You Post*

Knowing why you are online is the most crucial first step. Dermatologists can use social media to promote a practice, highlight academic work, educate patients, demonstrate clinical expertise, develop a professional brand, advocate for public health, or simply humanize the doctor–patient relationship. Every choice you make, including platform selection, posting frequency, tone, and visual style, is made easier when your goal is clear.[6,7]

[a] Department of Dermatology, University of Minnesota, Minneapolis, MN, USA; [b] Alluma Dermatology PLLC, Medina, MN, USA
* Corresponding author. Department of Dermatology, University of Minnesota, 516 Delaware Street S.E., Minneapolis, MN 55455.
*E-mail address:* olive550@umn.edu

Dermatol Clin 44 (2026) 589–598
https://doi.org/10.1016/j.det.2026.06.003

**Abbreviations**

| | |
|---|---|
| FDA | Food and Drug Administration |
| FTC | Federal Trade Commission |
| HIPAA | Health Insurance Portability and Accountability Act |

A purpose is not static. Every few months, you can assess whether your content is fulfilling both your audience's needs and your own career objectives by looking at analytics and engagement trends.[8] The following steps offer a simple framework for ongoing reassessment and course correction.

- Identify one primary purpose and one secondary purpose to guide content.
- Check to see whether this goal is reflected in your most recent posts.
- Reevaluate objectives every 3 months, changing course based on audience behavior and individual bandwidth.
- Use the following questions from **Fig. 1** to clarify your purpose:

## Pearl 2: Know Your Brand and Know Your Audience

Your professional identity becomes summarized in your brand. It reflects what you care about, how you communicate, and what your audience can expect from you. Expertise in hair loss, skin of color, cosmetic dermatology, chronic inflammatory disease, procedural dermatology, evidence-based skincare, or other dermatology-focused areas may be emphasized in by your brand. The most powerful brands maintain a consistent core identity while adjusting to each platform.[6]

Consider using a single account instead of separating your professional and personal profiles. Keeping everything in one place strengthens your brand identity, reduces confusion for your audience, and makes consistent engagement easier. Followers tend to connect best with a unified, authentic voice. Maintaining one account allows dermatologists to express personality while still being professional.[9] The following points outline practical considerations for defining a professional brand, selecting appropriate platforms, and aligning content with audience engagement.

- Write a one-sentence statement describing your professional brand.
- Choose platforms based on where your desired audience spends time.
- Use analytics to refine content types, tone, and posting frequency.
- When institutional policies allow, favor a single, professionally anchored account rather than multiple fragmented profiles.

### Writing an effective bio for a medical social media profile

On social media, you have only a few seconds to make a first impression. A strong bio helps people understand who you are, what you do, and why your voice matters. For dermatologists, clarity is essential. Your bio should communicate your professional identity, your clinical focus, and the value you offer, all in simple, approachable language.[10] An effective physician bio typically includes some or all of the following elements:

1. *Professional identity:* Degree and training level (eg, MD, DO, Resident, Fellow, Board-Certified Dermatologist).
2. *Clinical or educational focus:* Key areas of expertise that define your niche (eg, Acne, Hair Loss, Skin of Color, Evidence-Based Skincare).
3. *Purpose or value statement:* A concise description of what the audience can expect from your content (eg, "Education on hair health," "Helping you understand your skin.").
4. *Optional personal element:* A brief, humanizing detail that maintains professionalism while enhancing relatability (eg, coffee enthusiast, medical educator).

To support consistency across platforms, dermatologists can adapt the following template to

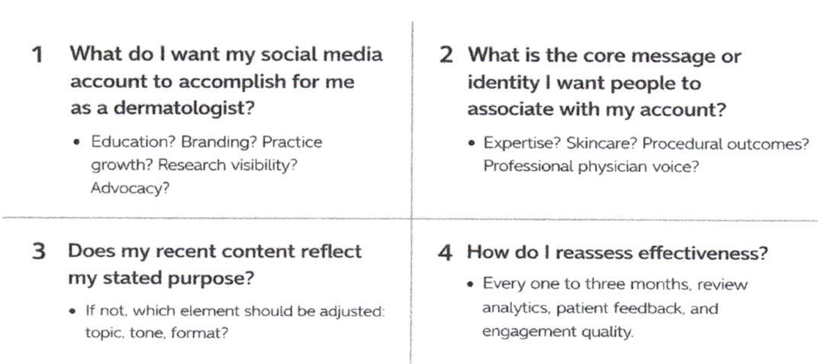


**Fig. 1.** Clarifying purpose in professional social media use. Key questions for intentional social media engagement.

fit their professional goals and areas of focus. **Fig. 2** illustrates a real-world example of how this framework can be applied in practice.

### *Example bio template for US physicians*

Full Name, Degree | Current Role | Institution | Location

Clinical Focus

Educational content only | Not medical advice

Link to Official Web site or Scheduling Portal

### *Choosing the right platform*

Understanding where patients spend their time online is important for dermatologists developing an effective digital strategy. Recent national survey data provide insights into social media platform use and demographic distribution.[11]

As shown in **Fig. 3**, YouTube and Facebook are the top platforms among US adults, with 84% using YouTube and 71% using Facebook. Instagram and TikTok occupy a strong middle tier and are particularly suited for visually driven dermatologic education and esthetic content because of their emphasis on short-form video and image-based storytelling.[11,12] These data help dermatologists prioritize where to invest their time, especially when managing multiple platforms is not feasible.

Age-based differences provide meaningful nuance in platform selection. As seen in **Fig. 4**, older adults report higher use of Facebook and YouTube. Dermatologists focusing on conditions that primarily affect older individuals may find better audiences on these platforms.[11]

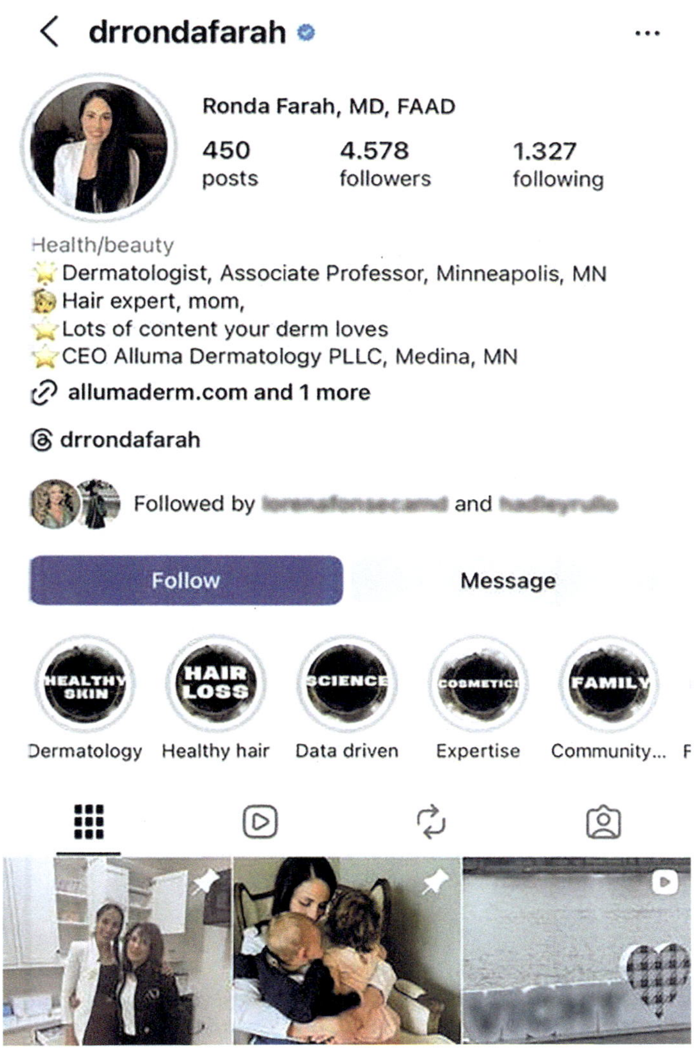


**Fig. 2.** Example of a purpose-aligned professional Instagram bio. (*From* Dr. Ronda Farah, Instagram post, @drrondafarah; with permission. Accessed on February 8th, 2026.)

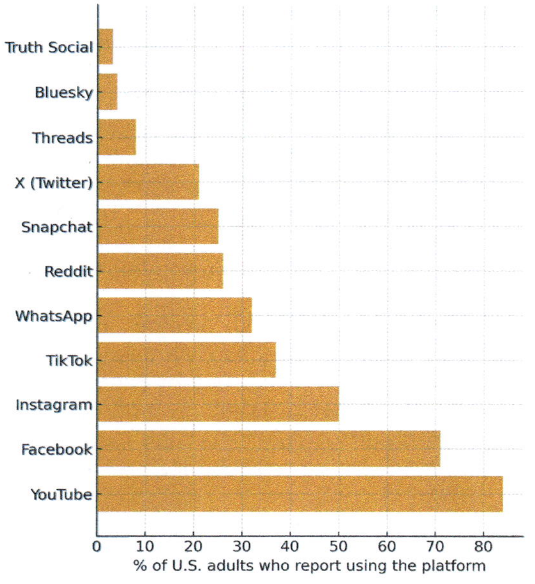


**Fig. 3.** Prevalence of social media use among US adults, 2025. Percentage of US adults who report using each platform. (Americans' Social Media Use 2025, by Jeffrey Gottfried and Eugenie Park. Pew Research Center, Washington, D.C. Nov 20, 2025. URL: https://www.pewresearch.org/internet/2025/11/20/americans-social-media-use-2025/.)

Beyond age, broader demographic variables influence how digital content is accessed and consumed. **Fig. 5** summarizes platform use across gender, race and ethnicity, education level, income, urbanicity, and political affiliation. Such trends suggest that effective communication tactics should consider demographic aspects of the community. Matching tone, language, and content style of communication with the diversity of the audience increases authenticity, inclusivity, and reach.[11]

In competitive practice environment, aligning platform strategy with demographic trends can influence referrals, patients recruitment, and positioning. Platform choice should align not only with general user prevalence but also with the demographic profile of the target patient population and the type of content being delivered.[9,13]

## *Pearl 3: Consistency Creates Trust and Visibility*

Consistency is key to sustainable success. Posting daily is often unrealistic for clinicians and can lead to burnout. Instead, focus on establishing a posting schedule that fits your routine.[14]

A visually consistent look also improves recognition. Similar backgrounds, lighting, and templates help build your style and enhance credibility. The tools such as content calendars and scheduling platforms facilitate your workflow and save time.[15]

While planned consistency forms the foundation of a strong online presence, selective flexibility also plays an important role. Live posting can

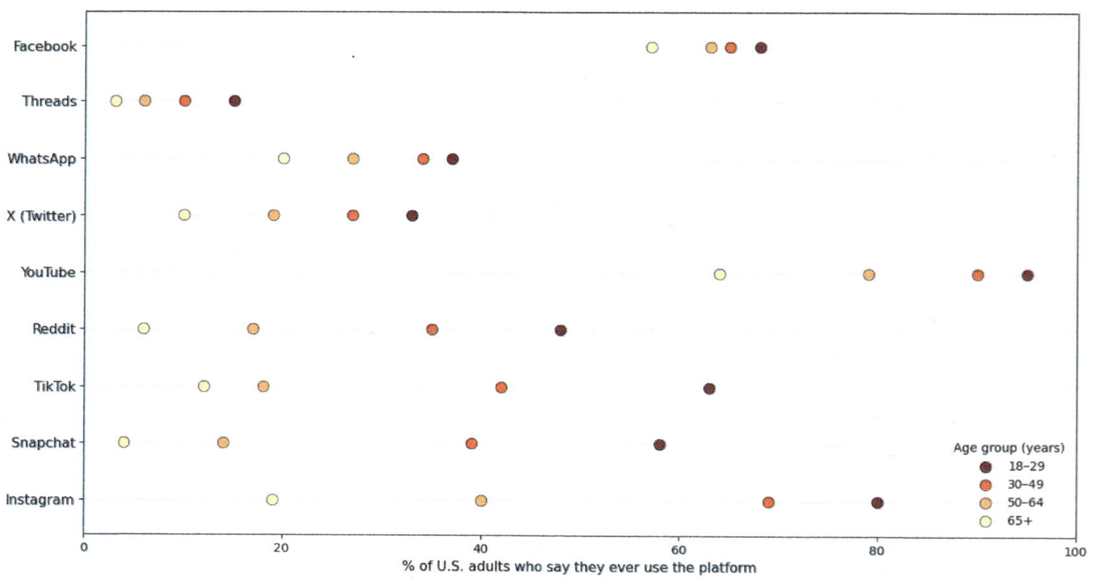


**Fig. 4.** Social media use by age group in the United States in 2025. Percentage of US adults within each age group who report ever using each platform. (Americans' Social Media Use 2025, by Jeffrey Gottfried and Eugenie Park. Pew Research Center, Washington, D.C. Nov 20, 2025. URL: https://www.pewresearch.org/internet/2025/11/20/americans-social-media-use-2025/.)

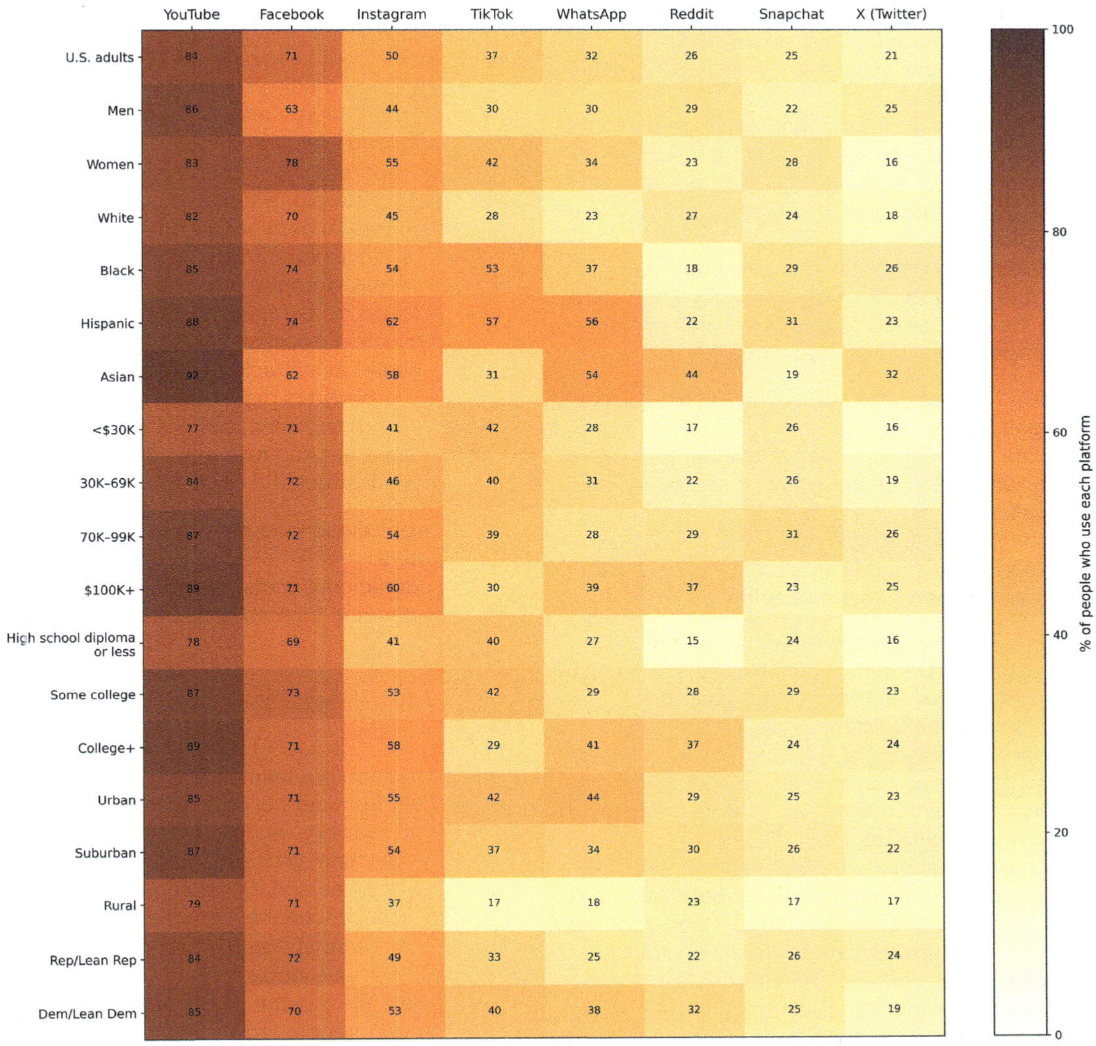


**Fig. 5.** Social media use across demographic groups in the United States, 2025. Percentage of US adults within each demographic category who report using each platform. (Americans' Social Media Use 2025, by Jeffrey Gottfried and Eugenie Park. Pew Research Center, Washington, D.C. Nov 20, 2025. URL: https://www.pewresearch.org/internet/2025/11/20/americans-social-media-use-2025/.)

boost engagement. Topics that relate to breaking news or something newsworthy usually perform better than pre-planned material. Audiences tend to pay more attention to current issues or trends. It is here that dermatologists take on a more journalistic role, quickly responding, providing clarity, and guiding the public discussion.[16] The following strategies outline practical ways to maintain consistency and flexibility in clinical social media use.

- Choose a posting frequency that is feasible for you, whether weekly, biweekly, or monthly.
- Use templates and presets to stick to one visual style.
- When possible, let trained staff handle filming or editing tasks to streamline your workflow.
- Record multiple pieces of content in one session to save time and keep your visuals consistent across posts.
- Share real-time insights when attending conferences, such as new research findings, emerging techniques, or clinical tips. This allows your audience to receive timely, relevant information while interest is high.

### *Pearl 4: Invest in Basic Production Quality*

Pictures and videos of excellent quality will make your video stand out and let people see the clinical details, techniques, or results. Poor lighting, distracting backgrounds, and unstable filming can make the most valuable information seem unprofessional.

Basic tools such as a ring light, tripod, and neutral filming space make a substantial difference. Make sure filming takes place in settings that guarantee patient privacy and professionalism.[17]

In addition to visual quality, clear audio is just as important for sustaining viewer attention and credibility. Several simple adjustments can substantially improve visual and audio quality:

- Use natural light or a ring light for even lighting.
- Film against simple, uncluttered backgrounds, like a plain white or neutral-colored wall.
- Stabilize videos using a tripod.
- Keep audio clean. A small clip-on microphone is an inexpensive and effective upgrade.

High-quality production extends beyond lighting and resolution. Dermatologists should responsibly represent diverse skin tones, hair types, ages, and genders in educational materials.[18] This increases inclusion, addresses the past exclusion of certain groups, improves diagnostic accuracy among viewers, and increases trust among those who have been marginalized.

Accessibility should also be prioritized as part of responsable production practices. Subtitles on all video content, readable fonts, high-contrast graphics, and descriptions for images help ensure that educational content remains acessible to individuals with hearing, visual, or cognitive limitations. These choices strengthen both professionalism and impact.[19]

### Pearl 5: Create Content Anyone Can Understand

Dermatology involves complex terminology, but social media communication needs to be accessible. Overly technical explanations can discourage viewers and lead to misunderstandings. Successful online dermatologists simplify complex ideas into simple language, use analogies to explain them, and provide visual examples when possible. Aim for clear, straightforward language in all posts.[19]

Storytelling through relatable clinical scenarios, common patient misconceptions, or practical tips helps maintain engagement and reinforce understanding. Captions and on-screen text further emphasize key messages, particularly for viewers who watch content without sound.[19]

### Pearl 6: Use Social Media as an Educational Platform

The use of social media provides a platform to correct misinformation, reduce fear, and share evidence-based recommendations. Dermatologists can address common concerns such as acne myths, steroid phobia, sunscreen safety, and other misconceptions. Educational series, weekly tips, "myth versus fact" posts, seasonal reminders, create structure and anticipation.[7]

For academic dermatologists, social media can disseminate publications, promote conferences, highlight departmental achievements, and engage trainees.[20] A consistent digital presence strengthens national visibility and enhances collaboration.[21] The following strategies can help turn educational intent into consistent, structured content:

- Highlight evidence-based information in simple ways.
- Pin educational posts for easy access.
- Use recurring themes or hashtags to organize content.

### Pearl 7: Protect Your Time, Boundaries, and Professionalism

Content creation is a learned skill, and dermatologists benefit from setting dedicated time aside for filming and editing. Avoid filming during clinic hours and maintain strict separation between clinical responsibilities and digital engagement.[17]

Professional boundaries should remain clear. Avoid giving personalized medical advice in comments. Always use documented consent for patient images. Be mindful of the Health Insurance Portability and Accountability Act (HIPAA) compliance in all filming locations.[17,22,23] The following safeguards help maintain professional integrity while sustaining a consistent digital presence:

- Dedicate a block of time monthly or weekly for content creation.
- Maintain strict privacy and confidentiality rules.
- Use clear disclaimers about general medical information.
- Keep in mind that anything you share online can remain there permanently.

More detailed ethical and regulatory considerations, including HIPAA, consent, and advertising rules, are outlined in Pitfall 7, and the Regulatory Considerations section.

### Pitfall 1: Setting Unrealistic Expectations

Daily posting is often not sustainable and leads to burnout. The skin experts will probably benefit more from a steady, manageable rhythm than from intense bursts of content followed by long absences. Growth should be viewed as a long-term process rather than a race against influencers.[23] To maintain sustainable growth:

- Choose a realistic posting frequency.
- Maintain a content "reserve" for busy months.
- Avoid comparing your growth to full-time creators.

### *Pitfall 2: Engaging in Emotionally Charged Comment Debates*

Comment sections can be unpredictable. Engaging in argumentative discourse rarely benefits the educational mission and may elevate conflict. Preparing standardized responses and anticipating common misconceptions creates clarity and saves time.[24]

If an online comment is particularly inflammatory, consider whether you would regret your response if it went viral. This thought exercise prevents reactionary posting.

The following strategies help preserve professionalism in public interactions:

- Before posting, imagine the worst comment or interaction that could follow. If you know it would be hard to handle publicly, choose not to post.
- Avoid reactive or emotional replies.
- Use standardized, planned responses to common misconceptions.
- Turn off comments selectively when necessary.

Similar considerations apply when responding to public reviews, where the stakes are often higher and responses are permanent. Online reviews on sites like Google, Yelp, Healthgrades, and RealSelf frequently influence patient decision-making.[25] Dermatologists, however, are limited by HIPAA and cannot confirm whether a reviewer is a patient or disclose any details of care. Emotional responses may unintentionally violate privacy or escalate tension.[24]

A safe strategy is to use neutral language that does not confirm a clinical relationship: "We are sorry to hear that your experience did not meet expectations. Please contact our office directly so we can address the concerns." This approach preserves professionalism while inviting offline resolution. In cases of widespread misunderstanding or negative response, pausing posting, consulting institutional communications teams, and issuing an explanation statement may be appropriate.[24]

### *Pitfall 3: Losing Authenticity*

Audiences respond to genuine, consistent voices. Imitating popular trends that do not fit your personality or clinical focus can feel forced, reducing trust.[26] Similarly, partnerships should align with your practice philosophy because your credibility is your most valuable asset. Always remain authentic and true to yourself:

- Post content aligned with personal practice patterns.
- Decline partnerships inconsistent with clinical values.
- Maintain a consistent voice across all platforms.

### *Pitfall 4: Not Collaborating*

Collaboration allows you to expand, and introduces your audience to new perspectives. Partnering with colleagues, institutions, photographers, and educators enhances creativity and builds community. Many dermatologists fail to collaborate due to unfamiliarity with digital networking, but even simple joint videos or shared graphics can increase visibility.[13] Consider ways to intentionally increase collaboration:

- *Co-create content for shared educational goals.* Join forces with others to build educational content that amplifies both your voices and your impact.
- *Stay connected with colleagues around the world.* Engage with their work and successes as well as their postings. When you support others, they naturally support you back, creating a cycle of collaboration.
- *Engage with professional societies or journals for structured initiatives* (eg, JAAD, JAMA Dermatology, AAD, ASDS, WDS, AHRS, BAD).
- *Engage with the brands and partners you already trust.* When you tag them in your posts, you open the door to visibility, connection, and often a reshared spotlight from the brand itself.

### *Pitfall 5: Misunderstanding Trends, Audio, or Platform Norms*

Trends can boost visibility, but their use must be intentional. Music with inappropriate lyrics, humor that feels unprofessional, or participation in formats that conflict with your brand can introduce reputational risk.[17] Dermatologists can adopt trend-inspired transitions or editing styles without adopting trends that misalign with their values. Approach trends with intention and discernment:

- Double-check audio before posting.

- Use trends selectively and thoughtfully.
- Prioritize professionalism over visibility.

### Pitfall 6: Correcting Misinformation Responsibly

Addressing misinformation is a crucial responsibility for dermatologists online, but it requires caution.[5] When correcting false claims, whether about sunscreen ingredients, hair loss treatments, or immunomodulators, avoid amplifying the misinformation by repeating it in detail or linking directly to misleading posts. Instead, summarize the misconception briefly, emphasize accurate evidence-based information, and offer practical guidance. Visual representation of the information, including "myth versus fact" graphics and brief explanatory videos, improve message clarity and reduce the risk of unintentionally amplifying the original misinformation.[27,28]

### Pitfall 7: Professional Boundaries and Ethical Responsibilities

Social media extends the physician-patient relationship into a public space, requiring dermatologists to find the right balance between accessibility and professionalism. Clinicians should avoid individualized medical advice in comments or direct messages, and all shared content must comply with advertising regulations and established standards of medical communication. Unlike influencers, physicians act within clearly defined frameworks, including HIPAA, professional ethics, institutional policies, medical board rules, and the broader obligation to maintain public trust.[17,22,23,29]

Maintaining patient confidentiality is central role to this process. When uncertainty exists, the safest approach is not to share anything. Disclaimers may support communication, but they should never be used as an excuse for ethical judgment or regulatory compliance.[17,22,23,29]

Beyond general professionalism, social media activity is subject to federal, state, and institutional oversight. Content involving medical products, procedures, sponsorships, or partnerships may be interpreted as promotional and must comply with Food and Drug Administration (FDA) and Federal Trade Commission (FTC) requirements, including balanced discussion of risks and benefits and clear disclosure of financial relationships.[17,30–32] State medical boards generally consider online activity an extension of professional conduct, even on personal accounts, and may monitor posts that could compromise patient privacy, or mislead the public.[29]

Comment sections and direct messages present a particular risk. Providing diagnoses, interpreting images, or offering individualized advice may unintentionally establish a physician–patient relationship with associated liability. A standardized response, such as "I cannot provide medical advice online, but I recommend scheduling a visit with a board-certified dermatologist," helps maintain boundaries while remaining supportive. If a message suggests urgent concern, clinicians may acknowledge the need for in-person evaluation but should avoid further triage or follow-up within social platforms.[17,29]

Clinical care, including teledermatology, must occur within secure, HIPAA–compliant systems that allow for consent, documentation, and follow-up. Social media platforms should not be

**Table 1**
**Ethical and professional safeguards for social media use in dermatology**

| Principle | What to Do |
|---|---|
| Protect Patient Identity | Never share identifiable patient information. Avoid faces, voices, tattoos, dates, locations, or background details that could reveal identity, even unintentionally. |
| Use Explicit, Platform-Specific Consent | Obtain written consent before posting any patient-related content. Clearly explain that social media posts may be permanent and widely shared. |
| Maintain Clinical Privacy | Film only in controlled environments. Ensure no background conversations, charts, names, or clinical details are visible or audible. |
| Educate Without Treating | Share general educational content only. Avoid case-specific advice, public diagnoses, or individualized recommendations; use clear disclaimers when appropriate. |
| Preserve Professional Boundaries and Credibility | Maintain respectful communication, avoid patient anecdotes, disclose conflicts of interest, and refrain from engaging in dual relationships or emotional online debates. |

used to diagnose, manage treatment, or communicate test results. Likewise, physicians working within institutions should clarify branding permissions, and content approval processes. When posting or editing is delegated, all contributors should receive HIPAA training, and clinicians should retain final review authority to ensure accuracy and compliance.[17,23]

Considering the complexity of regulatory and ethical expectations, having a simple reference point is helpful. **Table 1** offers a concise checklist to support safe, ethical, and professional social media use in dermatology.

## SUMMARY

Social media has become a natural extension of dermatologic practice, offering unique opportunities for education, advocacy, community building, and professional visibility. When used with intentionality, authenticity, and clear boundaries, social media strengthens trust and enhances patient understanding of dermatologic care. By embracing the pearls and avoiding the pitfalls outlined in this article, dermatologists can build sustainable digital identities that elevate the specialty and support the patients and communities they serve.

## CLINICS CARE POINTS

- Define a clear purpose and target audience before engaging on social media.
- Use a standardized physician bio and pin a few reference educational posts to establish credibility and set expectations.
- Share educational content only; avoid individualized medical advice in comments or direct messages.
- Establish clear boundaries through standardized policies for consent, comment moderation, and direct message responses.
- Ensure all content complies with ethical, institutional, and regulatory standards, including HIPAA, FDA, FTC, and medical board guidance.

## DISCLOSURE

The authors have nothing to disclose.

## REFERENCES

1. Amir M, Sampson BP, Endly D, et al. Social networking sites. JAMA Dermatol 2014;150(1):56.
2. Kang J, Szeto MD, Suh L, et al. Popular skin-of-color dermatology Social Media Hashtags on TikTok from 2021 to 2022: content analysis. JMIR Dermatol 2024;7. https://doi.org/10.2196/50408.
3. Szeto MD, Mamo A, Afrin A, et al. Social media in dermatology and an overview of popular social media platforms. Curr Dermatol Rep 2021;10(4):97–104.
4. Devjani S, Ezemma O, Fruechte S, et al. "Skinfluencers" versus dermatologists as creators of the top dermatology-related videos on TikTok. J Clin Aesthet Dermatol 2023;16(8):20–1.
5. Trepanowski N, Grant-Kels JM. Social media dermatologic advice: dermatology without dermatologists. JAAD Int 2023;12:101–2. Elsevier B.V.
6. Nguyen BM, Lu E, Bhuyan N, et al. Social media for doctors: taking professional and patient engagement to the next level. Fam Pract Manag 2020;27(1):14–9.
7. Cooper BR, Concilla A, Albrecht JM, et al. Social media as a medium for dermatologic education. Curr Dermatol Rep 2022;11(2):103–9. Springer.
8. Gonçalves A. Social media analytics strategy: using data to optimize business performance. New York (NY): Springer; 2017. https://doi.org/10.1007/978-1-4842-3102-9.
9. Ventola L. Social media and health care professionals: benefits, risks, and best practices. 2014. Available at: https://pmc.ncbi.nlm.nih.gov/articles/PMC4103576/. Accessed November 24, 2025.
10. Jain M, Malik P. Social media bio strategy and ideas for all platforms. Sprinklr. Available at: https://www.sprinklr.com/blog/social-media-bio/. Accessed November 25, 2025.
11. Gottfried J, Park E. Americans' social media use in 2025. Pew Research Center; 2025. Available at: https://www.pewresearch.org/internet/2025/11/20/americans-social-media-use-2025/. Accessed November 23, 2025.
12. Nigro AR, Osman A, Saal RC, et al. Information regarding dermatology as seen on the social media platform TikTok. JMIR Dermatol 2025;8. https://doi.org/10.2196/59597.
13. Mariwalla K. Social media. In: Dover Jeffrey S, Mariwalla K, editors. The business of dermatology. New York (NY): Thieme; 2020. p. 297–303.
14. Santos S, Gonçalves HM, Teles M. Social media engagement and real-time marketing: using net-effects and set-theoretic approaches to understand audience and content-related effects. Psychol Mark 2023;40(3):497–515.
15. Canva Team. What is brand identity? And how to create a strong brand. Canva 2025. Available at: https://www.canva.com/resources/brand-identity/. Accessed November 26, 2025.
16. Lu X, Balakrishnan K, Chan TJ, et al. The role of real-time engagement in shaping social media Check-In behavior: moderating effects of trust and peer influence. Brain Behav 2025;15(9). https://doi.org/10.1002/brb3.70887.

17. AMA. Professionalism in the use of social media. Opinion 2.3.2, AMA Code of Medical Ethics. 2017. Available at https://policysearch.ama-assn.org/policyfinder/detail/E-2.3.2%20?uri=%2FAMADoc%2FEthics.xml-E-2.3.2.xml (Accessed 25 November 2025).
18. Perlman KL, Williams NM, Egbeto IA, et al. Skin of color lacks representation in medical student resources: a cross-sectional study. Int J Womens Dermatol 2021;7(2):195–6. Elsevier Inc.
19. The public health communicators guide. Accessible Social Media for Public Health; 2024. Available at: https://publichealthcollaborative.org/wp-content/uploads/2024/05/202405015_PHCC_AccessibleSocial_v3-1.pdf. Accessed February 13, 2026.
20. Wojtara MS. Use of social media for patient education in dermatology: narrative review. JMIR Dermatol 2023;6. https://doi.org/10.2196/42609. JMIR Publications Inc.
21. Bressler MY, Grudnikoff E, Bressler Y, et al. Risks and benefits of using social media in dermatology: cross-sectional questionnaire study. JMIR Dermatol 2021;4(1):e24737.
22. The HIPAA journal. HIPAA social media guidelines. The HIPAA journal 2025. Available at: https://www.hipaajournal.com/hipaa-social-media/. Accessed January 21, 2026.
23. Federation of State Medical Boards. Physician Wellness and Burnout: Report and Recommendations of the Workgroup on Physician Wellness and Burnout. 2018. Available at: https://www.fsmb.org/siteassets/communications/draft-report-for-2018-hod—wellness-and-burnout.pdf.
24. Lewis W. Managing your online reputation. In: Dover JS, Mariwalla K, editors. The business of dermatology. New York (NY): Thieme; 2020. p. 309–14.
25. Henry M. Managing your online marketing and advertising your dermatology practice reputation. In: Dover JS, Mariwalla K, editors. The business of dermatology. New York (NY): Thieme; 2020. p. 320–6.
26. Zhong C, Chan H, Karamshuk D, et al. Wearing many (social) hats: how different are your different social network personae? Available at: http://arxiv.org/abs/1703.04791 (Accessed 25 November 2025), 2017.
27. Vraga EK, Bode L. Using expert sources to correct health misinformation in social media. Sci Commun 2017;39(5):621–45.
28. Chan MPS, Jones CR, Hall Jamieson K, et al. Debunking: a meta-analysis of the psychological efficacy of messages countering misinformation. Psychol Sci 2017;28(11):1531–46.
29. King P, Steingard S, Chaudhry H, et al, Social media and electronic communications. Federation of State medical records (FSMB), Available at: https://www.fsmb.org/siteassets/advocacy/policies/social-media-and-electronic-communications.pdf (Accessed 25 November 2025), 2019.
30. U.S. Food & Drug Administration (FDA). Basics of drug ads. 2015. Available at: https://www.fda.gov/drugs/prescription-drug-advertising/basics-drug-ads. Accessed November 26, 2025.
31. U.S. Food & Drug Administration (FDA). Drug advertising: a glossary of terms. 2020. Available at: https://www.fda.gov/drugs/prescription-drug-advertising/drug-advertising-glossary-terms. Accessed November 26, 2025.
32. Muzumdar S, Grant-Kels JM, Farshchian M. Ethics of social media marketing by dermatologists. J Am Acad Dermatol 2021;85(1):277–8. Mosby Inc.

# The Pearls and Perils of Social Media in Dermatology

Charles L. Dunn, MD[a,*], Sara Moghaddam, MD[b]

KEYWORDS

• Social media • Dermatology branding • Professionalism • Misinformation • Patient privacy
• Digital reputation • Ethics • Physician branding

## KEY POINTS

- Social media is one of the most influential communication tools for dermatologists, reaching billions worldwide as patients increasingly rely on it for health information.
- Strategic engagement can enhance patient education, professional networking, and brand development.
- The same platforms introduce ethical, legal, and reputational risks, including privacy violations, misinformation propagation, and commercial conflicts.
- Algorithmic incentives reward engagement rather than accuracy, requiring intentional counterbalancing by physicians.
- Structured safeguards, documentation practices, and clear personal policies are essential to mitigate predictable hazards.

## INTRODUCTION/BACKGROUND

The digital era has fundamentally altered how physicians communicate with patients, peers, and the public. The integration of social media into medical practice represents one of the most rapid cultural and technological shifts in modern health care communication. Within a relatively short period, digital platforms have transitioned from informal networking spaces to primary sources of health information, brand development, and professional discourse. Dermatology occupies a uniquely prominent position within this ecosystem due to the specialty's inherently visual diagnostic framework, public interest in cosmetic and medical skin concerns, and the relative accessibility of visual demonstration as an educational tool.

Historically, physician communication with the public occurred through institutional channels—academic publications, media interviews, and organized public health campaigns. Social media decentralizes these pathways, enabling individual clinicians to reach audiences numbering in the tens or hundreds of thousands without editorial gatekeeping. This democratization of voice is simultaneously empowering and destabilizing. It elevates physicians who engage thoughtfully while exposing those who participate impulsively to amplified reputational consequences.

The language of *pearls and perils* captures this duality. Social media is neither inherently beneficial nor inherently harmful; rather, it is a force multiplier. It magnifies professionalism when guided by intentionality and magnifies missteps when driven by impulsivity or commercial pressure. Understanding both dimensions is essential for dermatologists who seek to engage effectively in a landscape defined by speed, visibility, and permanence.

[a] Department of Dermatology, KCU / GME Consortium, Advanced Dermatology & Cosmetic Surgery, 1720 Dunlawton Avenue, Port Orange, FL 32127, USA; [b] Board Certified Dermatologist, Mohs Micrographic Surgeon, Delmarva Skin Specialists
* Corresponding author.
*E-mail address:* Charles.Luck.Dunn@gmail.com
Twitter: @Dunn.Derm.MD (C. L. D); @DrSaraMD (S. M)

Dermatol Clin 44 (2026) 599–606
https://doi.org/10.1016/j.det.2026.06.004
0733-8635/26/

| Abbreviations | |
|---|---|
| FSMB | Federation of State Medical Boards |
| FTC | Federal Trade Commission |

## PEARLS: THE STRATEGIC VALUE OF SOCIAL MEDIA ENGAGEMENT

### *Scale and Reach*

Global social media usage now exceeds *5 billion users worldwide*, representing much of the planet's population. In the United States, surveys consistently demonstrate that a substantial proportion of adults—particularly those under the age of 45 years—seek health information online prior to consulting a physician. Dermatologic conditions, because of their visual and often cosmetic impact, are disproportionately searched and discussed.

For dermatologists, this scale translates into

- *Unmatched audience access*
- *Rapid dissemination of evidence-based education*
- *Opportunity to counter misinformation*
- *Enhanced professional visibility*

Ignoring social media does not eliminate its influence; it merely cedes the space to nonexperts.

### *Patient Education and Public Health Impact*

Dermatology lends itself particularly well to visual education. Short videos explaining sunscreen application, acne myths, or early melanoma signs can reach hundreds of thousands of viewers within hours. Educational content often functions as *preventive medicine at scale*, reinforcing clinic-based counseling and promoting earlier care-seeking behavior.

Effective educational engagement can

- *Normalize dermatologic care*
- *Reduce stigma surrounding visible skin disease*
- *Improve adherence to treatment plans*
- *Encourage early detection of malignancy*

When executed thoughtfully, social media becomes an extension of the examination room rather than a substitute for it. The pearl in this vein lies not in volume of content but in clarity, consistency, and clinical integrity.

### *Professional Networking and Leadership*

Digital platforms function as decentralized professional conferences occurring continuously rather than in episodic manner as has historically been the case in professional medicine. Dermatologists can exchange clinical pearls, discuss emerging therapies, and engage in cross-disciplinary dialog. For early-career physicians and trainees, visibility within professional digital networks may facilitate mentorship opportunities that might otherwise be geographically or institutionally inaccessible.

Leadership development is also influenced by digital presence. Physicians who communicate clearly, responsibly, and consistently often become de facto public representatives of the specialty. This visibility can support advocacy efforts, promote specialty initiatives, and foster collective professional identity. However, leadership visibility simultaneously heightens accountability, underscoring the need for disciplined engagement.

### *Practice Growth and Brand Development*

From a business perspective, social media can powerfully influence patient acquisition and brand recognition. Importantly, studies support that the most effective professional branding is not overt advertisement but *credibility signaling*. Consistent educational messaging, demonstration of expertise, and professional demeanor build trust more sustainably than promotional content alone. The key lies in positioning oneself as a reliable source of evidence-based information rather than a commercial entity seeking attention. Authentic educational content often outperforms overt promotional messaging in fostering trust.

## KEYS TO EFFECTIVE ENGAGEMENT

Engaging effectively on social media requires the same intentionality, professionalism, and strategic planning that govern successful clinical practice and leadership. Visibility alone does not equate to influence, and influence without structure often leads to inconsistency or reputational drift. The most successful physician communicators approach digital participation not as spontaneous expression but as a deliberate extension of their professional identity and educational mission. Effective engagement, therefore, rests on a small set of repeatable principles that balance authenticity with credibility, accessibility with authority, and creativity with ethical restraint. When applied consistently, these principles allow dermatologists to leverage the reach of social media while preserving clarity of message, professional decorum, and long-term trust.

### *Clarify Purpose*

Every social media presence benefits from a clearly defined primary objective. Without intentional purpose, content tends to oscillate between education, promotion, humor, and personal expression in ways that dilute credibility and confuse audiences.

Common primary purposes include

- *Public education*—myth-busting, preventive health messaging, and awareness campaigns
- *Professional networking*—peer dialog, conference engagement, and academic collaboration
- *Practice development*—brand recognition, patient acquisition, and service visibility
- *Advocacy and leadership*—specialty representation, policy discussion, and public health initiatives

While multiple goals can coexist, identifying a dominant purpose guides tone, content selection, and posting frequency. Purpose functions as an editorial filter, ensuring that engagement remains coherent rather than reactive.

### *Identify the Target Audience*

Content that resonates with colleagues may be inaccessible or intimidating to patients, while patient-directed messaging may appear overly simplified to peers. Deliberate audience identification prevents misalignment between complexity, tone, and delivery style.

Typical audience categories include

- General public/patients
- Medical trainees
- Practicing colleagues
- Industry or policy stakeholders

Audience awareness influences vocabulary, depth of explanation, humor tolerance, and visual presentation. Effective communicators often visualize a single representative viewer when drafting posts, which promotes clarity and consistency.

### *Maintain Brand Consistency*

Professional branding in medicine is less about logos and more about *recognizable credibility*. Consistency in visual identity, messaging tone, and thematic focus reinforces trust and recall. Inconsistent branding can create cognitive dissonance, where the audience struggles to reconcile expertise with fluctuating presentation styles.

Key elements of consistency include

- Stable color palettes or visual motifs
- Predictable educational themes or series
- Uniform professional titles and credentials
- Alignment between online persona and in-person demeanor

Consistency does not preclude creativity; rather, it provides a framework within which creativity can occur without undermining authority.

### *Prioritize Quality over Frequency*

Algorithmic environments reward volume, but professional credibility is built through accuracy and substance. High-frequency posting without informational value risks audience fatigue and reputational dilution. Conversely, thoughtfully produced content—even at lower frequency—signals expertise and deliberation.

Quality-focused engagement emphasizes

- Evidence-based information
- Clear visual presentation
- Concise yet accurate explanations
- Avoidance of sensationalism for attention

A sustainable posting cadence that preserves accuracy is more beneficial than attempting to match platform velocity at the expense of professionalism.

### *Demonstrate Credentials Transparently*

In an environment where nonexperts often command large audiences, transparent credentialing serves as an important differentiator. Clearly displaying board certification, training background, and professional affiliations provides context for authority and reassures audiences regarding expertise.

Credential transparency may include

- Professional titles in profile descriptions
- Institutional affiliations when appropriate
- Disclosure of relevant certifications or subspecialties

This practice is not self-promotion; it is contextual clarification that allows audiences to evaluate information sources responsibly.

### *Engage with Trends Selectively and Intentionally*

Platform trends, viral formats, and cultural moments can expand reach, but indiscriminate participation may erode credibility or blur professional boundaries. Selective engagement ensures that trend adoption aligns with educational value and ethical standards rather than novelty alone.

Intentional trend engagement involves

- Evaluating whether the format supports accurate messaging
- Avoiding humor or satire that trivializes medical conditions

- Ensuring patient dignity and professionalism remain intact
- Adapting trends to educational objectives rather than mimicking them uncritically

The guiding principle is that trends should *serve the message*, not replace it. When trends are used as vehicles for evidence-based education rather than entertainment alone, they enhance reach without compromising professional identity (**Fig. 1**).

## PERILS: STRUCTURAL, BEHAVIORAL, AND PROFESSIONAL HAZARDS

In the setting of these inherent strengths, it is important to recognize that social media participation exposes dermatologists to a recurring set of vulnerabilities that differ in both origin and impact from traditional clinical interactions. These hazards generally fall into 3 interconnected domains: *structural hazards*, which arise from the design and incentive systems of digital platforms themselves; *behavioral hazards*, which stem from individual posting practices and boundary management; and *professional hazards*, which involve ethical, legal, and reputational consequences tied to physician identity and public trust. Algorithmic amplification and engagement-driven visibility pressures represent structural forces that shape what content is rewarded. Boundary erosion, oversharing, and emotional reactivity reflect behavioral risks that emerge from day-to-day digital conduct. Patient privacy breaches, implicit medical advice, and commercial conflicts constitute professional hazards with potential regulatory and medicolegal implications. Viewing these risks through a categorical framework allows dermatologists to anticipate and mitigate challenges proactively rather than responding only after harm has occurred. Let us look at a few of these individual risks a little closer.

### *Algorithmic Amplification and Sensationalism*

Social media algorithms are designed to maximize user engagement. Content that provokes strong emotional reactions—surprise, outrage, humor—receives preferential visibility. Knowing this may help with content creation, but it is important to recognize that clinical nuance, uncertainty, and evidence hierarchy are less compatible with rapid engagement metrics. Such a structural bias encourages oversimplification and sensationalism, potentially distorting patient expectations and professional standards.

### *Boundary Erosion and Identity Blurring*

Digital platforms collapse traditional distinctions between personal and professional identity. While authenticity fosters relatability, excessive informality may erode authority. Humor, lifestyle

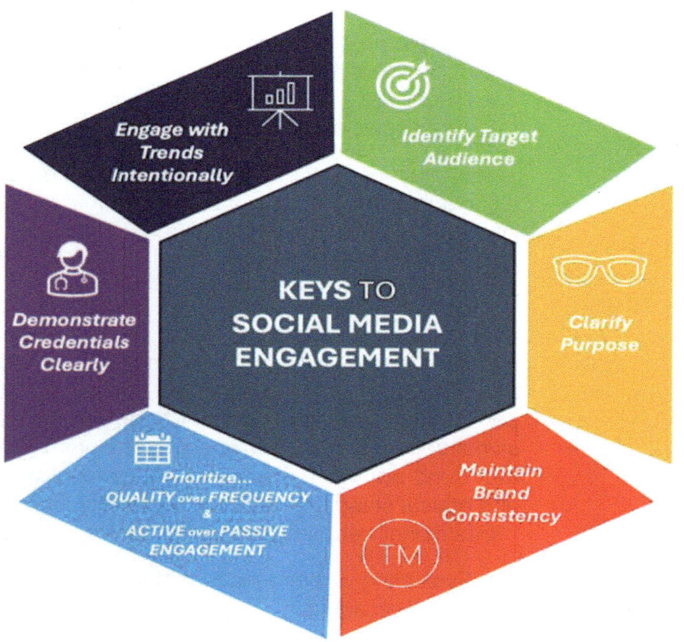
Engage with Trends Intentionally
Identify Target Audience
KEYS TO SOCIAL MEDIA ENGAGEMENT
Demonstrate Credentials Clearly
Clarify Purpose
Prioritize...
QUALITY over FREQUENCY
&
ACTIVE over PASSIVE ENGAGEMENT
Maintain Brand Consistency
TM

**Fig. 1.** Six keys to effective professional social media engagement.

disclosures, and personal commentary must be balanced against the expectation of professional decorum. The peril arises when relatability transitions into familiarity that undermines credibility or invites inappropriate expectations of accessibility.

### *Patient Privacy and Consent Failures*

Visual specialties face heightened risk of inadvertent patient identification.

*Tattoos,*
*Unique lesion patterns,*
*Background elements, and*
*Timestamps (either visual or verbal [ie, "a patient came to see me today..."])*

can reveal identity despite deliberate anonymization. The permanence and shareability of digital content magnify the consequences of even minor oversights. Consent must be explicit, documented, and revocable, yet even comprehensive consent does not eliminate ethical considerations regarding dignity and context.

### *Implicit Medical Advice and Liability*

Educational posts often function as individualized guidance despite disclaimers. *Context collapse*—where generalized advice is interpreted as personalized instruction—creates medicolegal vulnerability. Dermatologists must emphasize that digital content complements rather than replaces clinical evaluation, yet audience interpretation remains partially beyond the creator's control.

### *Commercial Conflicts and Perceived Bias*

Disclosures are an important component of brand-associated messaging, and the Federal Trade Commission (FTC) actively seeks to ensure commercial conflicts are visible and clear. Even when disclosures are provided, though, brand partnerships and sponsored content introduce reputational risk. Audiences may interpret financial relationships as endorsements, potentially eroding trust. Transparency is necessary but not sufficient; selectivity and alignment with professional values are equally critical.

### *Oversharing and Reputational Vulnerability*

Emotional venting, workplace commentary, or public disputes may persist indefinitely in searchable archives. The psychological toll of constant visibility—exposure to criticism, trolling, or performance pressure—can contribute to professional burnout. Digital restraint is both a reputational and mental health safeguard.

## RISK MITIGATION STRATEGIES

While one cannot simply remove these challenges, risk mitigation through specific safeguards can help. Risk mitigation in social media use is most effective when approached as a multilayered system rather than a series of isolated behaviors. Structural policies, behavioral guardrails, institutional alignment, psychological boundaries, and legal awareness function synergistically. When implemented together, these strategies convert social media from a reputational vulnerability into a controlled professional instrument. Importantly, many of these safeguards are extrapolated from broader digital professionalism and patient privacy standards that predate social media itself.

### *Structural Safeguards*

#### *Written social media policy*

A written personal or institutional social media policy acts as a precommitment mechanism, reducing impulsive posting and clarifying acceptable boundaries before ambiguity arises. Policies may be brief but should address at minimum

- Patient imagery and consent requirements
- Financial disclosures and sponsorship transparency
- Professional tone expectations
- Account separation guidelines
- Response protocols for criticism or misinformation

The American Medical Association and Federation of State Medical Boards (FSMB) both emphasize that physicians should maintain the same ethical standards online as offline, including confidentiality, professional decorum, and transparency regarding conflicts of interest. Written policies operationalize these expectations into daily behavior.[1–3]

#### *Account segmentation*

Maintaining distinct personal and professional accounts is not universally required but is strongly recommended in high-visibility specialties such as dermatology. Segmentation reduces identity blurring and limits cross-audience misinterpretation. Professional accounts should

- Use institutional or practice-aligned branding
- Avoid personal family or lifestyle content
- Maintain consistent educational tone

Personal accounts, even when private, should still assume eventual public visibility due to screenshot culture and digital permanence. The American College of Physicians has noted that privacy settings do not equate to confidentiality.

### *Standardized consent documentation*

Visual documentation presents unique challenges in dermatology. Written consent for digital dissemination should be

- Specific to social media use (not bundled into general treatment consent)
- Revocable at any time
- Securely stored and auditable
- Reaffirmed for reposts or secondary use

Even with consent, ethical considerations persist regarding dignity, power imbalance, and contextual framing. The Health Insurance Portability and Accountability Act establishes minimum legal standards, but professional societies consistently emphasize that ethical standards often exceed legal minimums.[4–9]

### *Scheduled posting and content calendars*

Impulsive posting is a leading contributor to reputational missteps. Structured scheduling systems encourage intentional messaging and reduce emotionally reactive communication. Content calendars also facilitate thematic planning around awareness months, public health campaigns, and educational series rather than sporadic output driven by algorithmic pressure.

## *Behavioral Safeguards*

### *The "delay principle"*

Instituting a deliberate delay—often 12 to 24 hours—before posting emotionally charged or controversial material substantially reduces reputational risk. Psychological research on decision-making demonstrates that emotional arousal narrows cognitive framing and increases risk-taking behaviors. The delay principle allows for cognitive recalibration and peer consultation when needed.

### *Avoidance of real-time clinical metrics*

Posting procedural counts, operative durations, or revenue-adjacent metrics can invite regulatory scrutiny, misinterpretation by the public, and accusations of commercialization. The FSMB has cautioned that online statements reflecting clinical productivity or superiority claims may be interpreted as advertising or misleading representation.[2] Broad, qualitative descriptors are preferable to quantitative disclosures.

### *Framing education broadly rather than individually*

Educational posts should emphasize generalizable principles rather than individualized recommendations. Even when disclaimers are present, audiences frequently generalize case-specific advice to personal conditions—a phenomenon known as *context collapse*. Broad framing reduces liability exposure and reinforces the distinction between education and medical advice.

### *Periodic content audits*

Quarterly or biannual reviews of archived posts help identify outdated recommendations, evolving evidence bases, or potentially problematic phrasing. Digital permanence means that posts remain searchable long after publication. Content audits function as retrospective quality assurance analogous to chart review or peer review processes in clinical practice.

## *Professional Alignment and Continuing Education*

### *Specialty society guidance*

Alignment with professional society guidance provides defensible standards and reduces ambiguity. Dermatology-specific initiatives, such as organized campaigns promoting board certification recognition and patient education, offer structured messaging frameworks that reduce improvisational risk. Society affiliation also lends credibility and mitigates perceptions of self-promotion.

### *Peer consultation*

A second-reader model for high-visibility or potentially controversial posts mirrors established academic practices. Informal peer review prior to publication can identify unintended interpretations, tone inconsistencies, or privacy concerns that may be invisible to the original author.

### *Continuing education in digital professionalism*

Digital professionalism is an evolving competency. Formal continuing medical education modules addressing online communication, misinformation management, and privacy compliance enhance adaptive awareness. Studies examining professionalism curricula in medical training demonstrate improved boundary recognition and reduced online misconduct when explicit instruction is provided.

## *Psychological and Boundary Safeguards*

### *Time boundaries and cognitive load management*

Unrestricted engagement with social media increases cognitive load and emotional fatigue. Establishing defined time limits for platform interaction preserves mental health and reduces compulsive monitoring behaviors. Physician burnout literature increasingly identifies digital overload as a contributing factor to professional exhaustion.

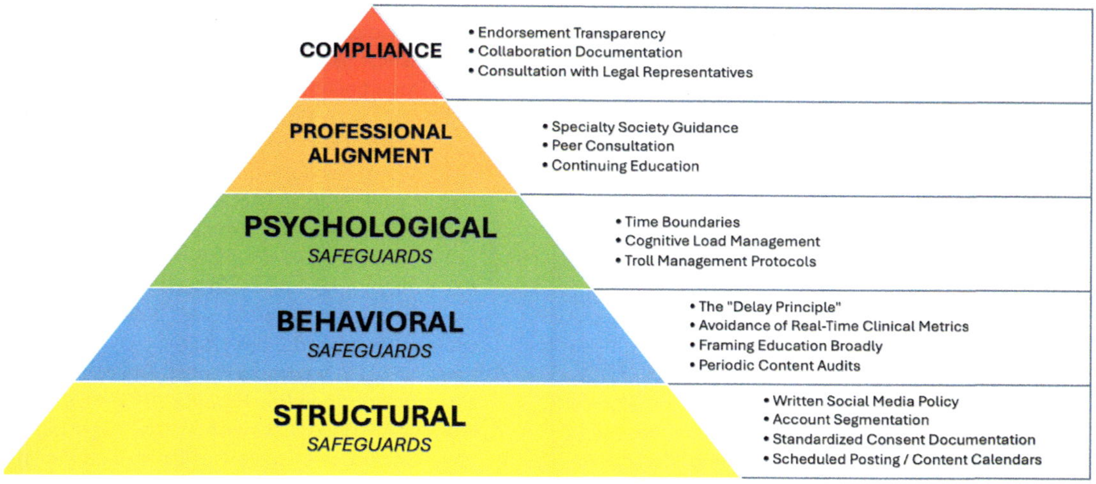


Fig. 2. Hierarchical pyramid of recommended safeguards for dermatologists engaging with social media. The model organizes protective measures into five ascending layers: foundational structural safeguards (written social media policies, account segmentation, standardized consent documentation, and scheduled posting/content calendars); behavioral safeguards (the "Delay Principle," avoidance of real-time clinical metrics, broad framing of educational content, and periodic content audits); psychological safeguards (time boundaries, cognitive-load management, and troll-management protocols); professional alignment (specialty-society guidance, peer consultation, and continuing education); and, at the apex, compliance measures (endorsement transparency, collaboration documentation, and consultation with legal representatives). The structure emphasizes that higher-level professional and regulatory protections rest on solid operational and personal foundations.

#### *Troll management protocols*

Predefined response strategies—such as selective nonengagement, templated responses, or comment moderation—prevent escalation. The goal is not censorship but preservation of professional tone and avoidance of reactive discourse. Emotional restraint maintains credibility and protects psychological well-being.

### *Legal and Compliance Awareness*

#### *Advertising and endorsement transparency*

The FTC requires clear and conspicuous disclosure of material connections between endorsers and commercial entities.[10] Even unpaid product mentions may be interpreted as endorsements if professional authority is implied. Transparent disclosure language protects both physician and audience.

#### *Documentation of sponsored collaborations*

Written agreements, disclosure statements, and archival documentation of partnerships provide legal insulation. These records should be retained similarly to other professional contracts.

#### *Consultation with compliance or legal teams*

Physicians affiliated with academic institutions or multiphysician practices should align social media activity with institutional compliance policies. Early consultation prevents retroactive corrective action and reinforces organizational trust (Fig. 2).

## SUMMARY

In summary, social media is neither inherently advantageous nor inherently detrimental to dermatologic practice. Its impact is determined by intentionality, professionalism, and structural safeguards. The *pearls*—education, networking, leadership visibility, and brand development—are substantial and increasingly indispensable in modern medicine. The *perils*—privacy breaches, misinformation, oversharing, commercial conflicts, and reputational permanence—are equally predictable. Dermatologists who engage with strategic clarity, ethical awareness, and robust mitigation frameworks can transform social media from a liability into a leadership asset.

## CLINICS CARE POINTS

- Define a primary purpose before posting; consistent educational messaging builds greater trust than unfocused or predominantly promotional content.
- Obtain explicit, social media–specific consent before sharing patient images, even when photographs appear de-identified.
- Prioritize evidence-based accuracy over viral engagement; algorithms reward attention, but credibility depends on scientific integrity.

- Maintain separate professional and personal accounts to preserve boundaries, reduce audience confusion, and protect your digital reputation.
- Treat every post as permanent and public; routinely audit older content to ensure accuracy, professionalism, and compliance.

## DISCLOSURE

The authors have nothing to disclose.

## REFERENCES


1. American Medical Association. Code of Medical Ethics Opinion 2.3.2: Professionalism in the Use of Social Media. Chicago (IL): American Medical Association, Available at: https://code-medical-ethics.ama-assn.org/ethics-opinions/professionalism-use-social-media (Policy Finder) (Accessed 6 July 2026).
2. Federation of State Medical Boards. Model Policy Guidelines for the Appropriate Use of Social Media and Social Networking in Medical Practice. Euless (TX): Federation of State Medical Boards; 2012 (reaffirmed/updated guidance available online). Available at: FSMB Social Media and Electronic Communications Policy (Federation of State Medical Boards) (Accessed 6 July 2026).
3. Farnan JM, Snyder Sulmasy L, Worster BK, et al. Online medical professionalism: patient and public relationships. Ann Intern Med 2013;158(8):620–7.
4. U.S. Department of Health and Human Services, Office for Civil Rights. HIPAA for Professionals. Washington (DC): U.S. Department of Health and Human Services; 2024. Available at: HIPAA for Professionals (HHS.gov) (Accessed 6 July 2026).
5. American Academy of Dermatology Association. Social Media and Professionalism Resources. Rosemont (IL): American Academy of Dermatology Association; Available at: AAD Social Media Resources (Accessed 6 July 2026).
6. Lerner JS, Li Y, Valdesolo P, et al. Emotion and decision making. Annu Rev Psychol 2015;66:799–823.
7. Marwick AE, Boyd D. I tweet honestly, I tweet passionately: twitter users, context collapse, and the imagined audience. New Media Soc 2011;13(1):114–33.
8. Chretien KC, Tuck MG, Simon M, et al. A digital professionalism curriculum for medical students. Acad Med 2015;90(6):753–60.
9. Shanafelt TD, Dyrbye LN, West CP. Addressing physician burnout: the way forward. JAMA 2017;317(9):901–2.
10. Federal Trade Commission. Guides Concerning the Use of Endorsements and Testimonials in Advertising. 16 CFR Part 255. Washington (DC): Federal Trade Commission; Available at: FTC Endorsement Guides (16 CFR Part 255) (Accessed 6 July 2026).

# Leadership During Times of Crisis

George J. Hruza, MD, MBA[a,b,c,*]

**KEYWORDS**

• COVID-19 • AAD • Leadership • Crisis • Strategy

**KEY POINTS**

- Effective crisis leadership relies on 14 key attributes: compassion, information, decisiveness, organization, focus, teamwork, delegation, consensus, communication, adaptability, relationships, trustworthiness, confidence, and strategy.
- Servant leadership was central: prioritizing members and patients over personal agendas while maintaining transparent, trustworthy communication throughout the pandemic.
- These principles can be applied to public service, where relationships, trustworthiness, communication, strategic focus, and adaptability prove especially valuable in legislative work.

*With the American Academy of Dermatology's 2020 Annual Meeting 3 weeks away, we have been closely monitoring developments with coronavirus disease discovered in 19 (COVID-19), commonly known as the coronavirus. The American Academy of Dermatology (AAD) is taking COVID-19 very seriously and is fully engaged and prepared to host a successful Annual Meeting in Denver. Currently, registration remains strong with roughly 14,400 registrants. While the CDC advises that the immediate risk from COVID-19 is low, the AAD is taking all necessary precautions to ensure the health and safety of attendees.*

*—Feb. 28, 2020, Elizabeth Usher, AAD Executive Director.*

This was the calm before the storm. The next few weeks and months tested the survival skills of the entire world and, in a local microcosm, our patients, dermatologists, and the Academy. Very few people alive in 2020 had experienced the last pandemic in 1918 to 1919, where 50 million people died. I was AAD President at the time. It fell to me to do my best to help our members and their patients navigate the pandemic and make sure that the Academy would survive to fight another day.

## WHAT ATTRIBUTES MAKE AN EFFECTIVE LEADER IN TIMES OF CRISIS?

When a crisis hits, especially one with no precedent like COVID-19, there are several characteristics or behaviors that I found helpful to get us through the pandemic.

## COMPASSION

*Leadership is about empathy. It is about having the ability to relate to and connect with people for the purpose of inspiring and empowering their lives.*

*—Daniel H. Pink*[1]

[a] Department of Dermatology, St. Louis University, St Louis, MO, USA; [b] Representative, Missouri State House; [c] Schweiger Dermatology Group, 1001 Chesterfield Parkway East, Suite 101, Chesterfield, MO 63017, USA
* Department of Dermatology, St. Louis University, St Louis, MO.
*E-mail address:* ghruza@gmail.com
Twitter: @george.hruza
Instagram: @george.hruza
Facebook: https://www.facebook.com/george.hruza/

Dermatol Clin 44 (2026) 607–612
https://doi.org/10.1016/j.det.2026.05.004

| Abbreviation | |
|---|---|
| AAD | American Academy of Dermatology |

In February 2020, I started getting emails from friends and colleagues about the looming pandemic. They were concerned about someone catching the virus at the meeting. Initially, they suggested various precautions we should be taking. As the days went on, the emails became more urgent, asking me to consider canceling the meeting. Finally, some were pleading for me to cancel the meeting lest some attendee might die from catching the virus at the Denver meeting. I made sure to hear out all who contacted me and responded with reassurance that I heard them and would take their concerns into consideration. I stayed away from being alarmist and stoking panic. This allowed their stress level to go down and allowed me to assess the pros and cons of what we should do about the meeting.

## INFORMATION

*In God we trust. All others bring data.*
*—W. Edwards Deming*[2]

Before making any decision, I made sure that we had all the information we could gather about COVID infectivity, the value of measures such as masks and distancing, as well as the incidence of the virus in Denver, the meeting venue. We also needed to know the financial implications of canceling the meeting, as our annual meeting generated more than 40% of our annual revenue. What nonrefundable costs would we be exposed to? Was there any insurance to offset those costs? If we had a total loss, no refunds, no revenue, no insurance, the Academy would be at major risk to its financial stability. The excellent AAD staff did a yeoman's job to get us the information. I communicated with other organizations that were planning to hold large meetings. I spoke with the President of the American Academy of Orthopedic Surgeons. She insisted that their meeting would go on come what may. They canceled their meeting a few days later.

## DECISIVENESS

*In any moment of decision, the best thing you can do is the right thing. The worst thing you can do is nothing.*
*—Theodore Roosevelt*[3]

Once all the information was analyzed, it was time to decide. We were getting very close to the exhibitors shipping their materials to Denver. Time was of the essence to make a decision. We determined that many universities would not allow their staff to attend and speak at any meetings, which meant that we were rapidly losing enough speakers to put on a quality meeting. The AAD had pandemic insurance, and hotels and airlines were willing to make various accommodations. With this information in hand, 2 weeks before the meeting, I called a Board of Directors meeting, presented the facts, and my recommendation that we cancel the meeting. All attendees would get a full refund of their registration fees and hotel deposits. The airlines would keep the value of tickets for future use without penalty (in 2020, airlines still charged $150 to change plane tickets). Our pandemic insurance would kick in as we could not put on a quality meeting. The insurance covered most of the nonrefundable costs and lost revenue. I presented our recommendation that the meeting be canceled. After a robust discussion, the Board of Directors approved my recommendation. This decision was made 2 weeks before the start of the meeting (just 1 week after the quote in the introduction). It was made 1 day before the exhibitors were to ship their exhibition materials. Phew! A week later, the Denver Convention Center shut down—no meetings allowed. We immediately communicated our decision to the membership, offering support in unwinding their plans to come to Denver.

## ORGANIZATION

*A good system shortens the road to the goal.*
*—Orison Swett Marden*[4]

The AAD staff immediately got to work to organize all the logistics of issuing refunds to 14,400 attendees and exhibitors, pulling together thousands of pieces of information for our insurance claim. Work also began to put together a virtual meeting, which was a very novel concept at the time. We wanted to make sure that our members did get access to important clinical continuing medcial education (CME).

## FOCUS

*If you spend too much time thinking about a thing, you'll never get it done.*
*—Bruce Lee*[5]

On March 16, 2020, the White House announced 15 days to slow the spread as COVID-19 incidence was taking off. It was clear that we would need to deal with it for an extended period of time. As my last act as AAD President, I set up the COVID-19 Task Force to focus on helping our members navigate the pandemic in their professional lives. As we were shut down, I was able to become laser-focused on helping our members navigate the pandemic. I knew that there was nothing I could do about the havoc COVID-19 was wreaking across the world. Stressing over that could have been paralyzing. Instead, I focused on what I could have a positive impact on: the Academy, our members, and our patients.

## TEAMWORK

*The strength of the team is each individual member. The strength of each member is the team.*

*—Phil Jackson*[6]

In setting up the COVID-19 Task Force, I made sure to include dermatologists with varied backgrounds, including academic, private practice, and infectious disease expertise. It was already clear that the pandemic was becoming politicized. I made sure to include members across the political spectrum. I wanted assertive individuals who would be willing to share their unvarnished opinions. I wanted to avoid groupthink (remember the Challenger O-rings?). I have found that teams with a range of opinions and experiences tend to make better decisions. The information from the Centers for Disease Control (CDC), Centers for Medicare and Medicaid Services (CMS), Small Business Administration (SBA), and other governmental agencies was coming fast and furious. Changes in rules, guidelines, and directives came almost hourly. Our Task Force started out with calls almost daily, and later weekly for many months.

## DELEGATION

*If you want to do a few small things right, do them yourself. If you want to do great things and make a big impact, learn to delegate.*

*—John C. Maxwell*[7]

There was no way one individual could keep on top of the massive information output from the myriad government agencies and the scientific community (this was before AI had become a thing). I had the AAD staff keep up with the missives coming from the various sources on COVID-19. They organized and summarized the information. Delegating as many tasks as possible allowed the Task Force to focus on informed strategic and tactical decisions.

## CONSENSUS

*A genuine leader is not a searcher for consensus but a molder of consensus.*

*—Martin Luther King Jr.*[8]

As the pandemic exploded through the population, hospitals in some regions (especially New York City) filled up with COVID-19 patients with respiratory compromise. Elective procedures and hospital admissions were stopped with federal guidelines and state regulations and laws to make sure there would be capacity to take care of COVID-19 patients. Some states expanded these bans on elective procedures to ambulatory surgery centers and even physician offices, at risk of disciplinary action on their physician license. In Missouri, I was able to successfully advocate for no government restrictions on office-based practice, as those restrictions seemed to be a misreading of the federal guidance. There was no concern about capacity in medical offices. Going to the physician's office had no different risk than going to the grocery store, and with the significant precautions we recommended be taken, the risk of infection there was significantly lower. Our Task Force had a lively discussion as to what we should recommend for taking care of dermatology patients in our offices. We weighed the potential risk of COVID-19 patient exposure in our office versus providing needed dermatology patient care. I made sure that the Task Force had all the known factual information stripped of the political spin that had, by then, crept into COVID-19 discussion. We ultimately achieved consensus recommending that in-person patient visits should be limited to patients with urgent and emergency issues, to be determined by the physician's clinical judgment with appropriate precautions to minimize the risk of in-office transmission of the virus. Of course, any state restrictions would take precedence.

## COMMUNICATION

*The art of communication is the language of leadership.*

*—James Humes*[9]

Information on the pandemic was coming in fast and furious. The Task Force worked through the often cryptic, vague, and constantly changing guidance from the various government agencies and the scientific community and made sure to share factual information with our members in a timely manner. We developed a communication strategy by setting up a portion of the AAD website to house the key information we had. We sent out member alerts regularly, often within hours of new critical information becoming available. We laid out the proper precautions and practices that should be taken to continue operating safely, including proper N-95 mask use, examining patients in the examination room, all surfaces cleaning protocols, and many others. We developed recommendations for offering telemedicine to patients and educated our members on the ins and outs of telemedicine. We adapted the ever-changing CDC guidelines on COVID-19 exposed or infected staff for the dermatologist's office. For practice financial sustainability, we gave members guidance as to accessing PPP loans and subsequently loan forgiveness, SBA emergency loans and grants, and payroll tax refunds. I and AAD staff fielded calls and emails from members regarding accessing all the government help available. My practice would have gone belly up without help from the PPP program. Being in the thick of it with our members gave me a better understanding of where they were and how we could help them navigate the process.

## ADAPTABILITY

*It is not the strongest of the species that survives, nor the most intelligent. It is the one that is most adaptable to change.*

—*Leon C. Meggison*[10]

As the government agencies kept changing their recommendations and as our understanding of COVID-19 improved, we had to keep adapting our recommendations, sometimes on a daily basis. Paycheck Protection Program (PPP) loans were available only for salaries and not for other expenses, then PPP money was available for rent expenses. PPP money was not available for newer practices that did not have a track record—until they were. One could not access PPP money as well as the payroll tax credit—until they were. It is the same SBA emergency credits and loans. This applied to precautions against infection such as regular surgical masks or even cloth masks were thought to be recommended until it became clear that only N-95 masks worn properly and continuously would provide some protection against infection. We shared our recommendations with our members in real time to make sure they had the most up-to-date information to make the most appropriate decisions for their practices and their patients.

## RELATIONSHIPS

*Personal relationships are the fertile soil from which all advancement, all success, all achievement in real life grows.*

—*Ben Stein*[11]

The AAD has cultivated relationships with many stakeholders in the executive and legislative branches of the federal government. As issues came up for our member practices dealing with COVID-19, we were able to leverage our relationships to get modifications and relief for our members. Getting major relaxation of telemedicine regulations to allow many versions of telemedicine including audio only and across state lines along with reimbursement levels on par with in-office visits was a major positive result of our (and organized medicine's) strong relationships with stakeholders and robust advocacy. On the business side of the equation, we were able to successfully advocate to simplify the application process for the various government support programs. Our advocacy helped expand access to both the PPP loans and the payroll tax credit programs simultaneously. I found developing personal relationships with the Task Force members helped to build trust and confidence in each other, making this a high-performing team with minimal conflict.

## TRUSTWORTHINESS

*Trust is the emotional glue that binds followers and leaders together.*

—*Warren G. Bennis*[12]

One of the early victims of the COVID-19 pandemic was trust in our elected officials and the government at large. Due to the fear of the unknown, many *experts* were coming up with various recommendations of dubious scientific value, such as COVID-19 *cures*. Responsible public health officials made statements of fact about appropriate precautions one should take without having the supporting evidence. Think about the recommended 6-foot separation between individuals, which later was determined to have limited, if any, benefit in reducing infection rates due to the highly infectious nature of the virus through aerosols as well as droplets (like the common cold virus spreads). The benefits of cloth and surgical masks that turned out to not be helpful in reducing infections. Stating these and other recommendations that turned out to not be accurate undermined the public's trust in public officials and the underlying science. In our Task Force, we made sure to only put out factual information, without spin, and included caveats about the strength of our recommendations. When new information arose, we immediately updated our members and updated our COVID-19 website. If people lose trust, they tend to not accept new information from that source. Witness the skepticism that COVID-19 vaccinations were met with and the many conspiracy theories that circulated about them and COVID-19. This damage to trust in science has persisted since the pandemic.

## CONFIDENCE

> *A good leader inspires people to have confidence in the leader; a great leader inspires people to have confidence in themselves.*
>
> *—Eleanor Roosevelt.*

The pandemic presented to many as an existential crisis, leading to stress and, for some, overwhelming anxiety that led to making rash decisions or having apocalyptic thoughts. Some were so overwhelmed as to not be able to take action. I found projecting confidence with humility to our members and Task Force provided reassurance that we have their back and are working overtime to help them get through the pandemic. This had to be confidence based on knowledge and willingness to express what we didn't know as well as what we knew with certainty. Confidence and trust go hand in hand. I stuck to what I knew: how to navigate the byzantine government system for the various regulatory requirements such as telemedicine expansion and shifting PPP procedures and steps to reduce risk of transmission in the office. I stayed away from talking about the various proposed medical treatments for COVID-19 such as ivermectin, hydroxychloroquine, and azithromycin. All 3 seemingly promising treatments that turned out to be not so helpful in the final analysis. This allowed us to maintain trust and confidence in our other actionable advice.

## STRATEGY

> *The essence of strategy is choosing what not to do.*
>
> *—Michael Porter*[13]

To be successful, an overarching strategy, vision, and mission have to be kept in mind, and all steps we take are to be held up to the short-term and long-term strategy of the Academy. As far as COVID-19, I viewed the short-term strategy as making sure that the Academy would do no harm by avoiding contributing to the spread of the virus to attendees and exhibitors and the public at large at the annual meeting. Second was that the Academy would survive the pandemic financially to fight another day. The long-term strategy is to continue supporting our members to provide high-quality accessible dermatologic care to our patients. We met our short-term goals through the pandemic with the help of AAD staff, the Board of Directors, and the COVID-19 task force. My successors at the helm of the Academy continue to execute admirably on the long-term strategy.

## SERVANT LEADERSHIP

> *Leadership is not about being in charge. Leadership is about taking care of those in your charge.*
>
> *—Simon Sinek*

To be successful leading a nonprofit institution such as the AAD, one has to always bring it back to the members. What is important to them? How can we help them achieve their goals? The role of AAD President is that of a servant leader. Personal agendas have no place in such a position. How the AAD navigated through the COVID-19 pandemic was a case study of servant leadership. All our efforts at the Academy were focused on helping our members get through the pandemic to be able to continue taking care of their patients once the crisis had passed. I found leading the COVID-19 Task Force the most gratifying purposeful professional activity that I have had the honor to be part of. Most dermatologists already practice servant leadership in their practices. We take care of our patients, keeping them front and center and doing everything we can to help them get the care they need. I certainly hope that some of the readers of this article will step up to lead the Academy in the same vein.

## PUBLIC SERVICE

During my experience with COVID-19 at the helm of the AAD and the COVID-19 Task Force, and the subsequent M-pox Task Force, I was able to apply several the leadership attributes navigating those crises. I realized that public service would be an opportunity to expand my support beyond dermatology to all the residents in Missouri. I ran for and won my race to the Missouri State House. Even though all the attributes listed are helpful in that leadership role, 5 stand out: *relationships, trustworthiness, communication, strategic focus*, and *adaptability*.

*Relationships* are the coin of the realm in the legislature. Helping other legislators with legislation that is important to them, getting to know them personally and, for me as a dermatologist, helping out with any skin complaints builds relationships. This becomes a virtuous cycle of supporting each other's legislation to get it over the finish line.

In politics, *trustworthiness* is a rare and valuable commodity. Honesty and truthfulness is a recipe for success. I had a bill in front of the Rules Committee that the Chair had some issues with and would not bring it up for a vote. I promised him that I would work in good faith to amend the bill on the floor. We agreed on a handshake, and he voted the bill out of the committee and, as promised, I put the amendment onto my bill on the floor. This would not have been possible if there was a lack of trust in my word by the Chair.

Constituent *communication* and assistance are key for reelection. The voters that put me into office need to know that I am keeping their concerns top of mind at all times. It is very easy to get distracted by the activity in the legislature with more than 2000 bills filed each year.

I find being *strategically focused* on the big picture and what I and my caucus want to accomplish keeps me grounded and effective. Each year I set a main goal to achieve. The first year we were able to eliminate the Missouri state capital gains tax, the second year I am close to passing a K-20 Jewish public student safety bill, next year will be the elimination of the state income tax in a revenue-neutral way to change Missouri's economic trajectory in a positive direction.

Missouri's legislature consists of 163 representatives and 34 senators. Each one has their own ideas as to the best thing to do to help move Missouri forward. As such, one has to be willing to *adapt* to the changing situation on the ground as political winds shift and alliances in the legislature shift. It is important to be a good listener as the other legislators come from very different backgrounds than my own. In the Missouri legislature there are only 2 physicians. I have found the experience purposeful and meaningful. Public service is not for everyone, but for those that do take the plunge they will find it very worthwhile.

## CLINICS CARE POINTS

When encountering a crisis situation in your practice, we have found the following steps to be helpful:

- Get as much information as possible by leveraging your relationships with those you trust.
- Gather consensus from stakeholders as to what actions they might recommend.
- When you make a decision as to the course of action, present it with confidence.
- Communicate your decision and plan of action with compassion.
- Focus on executing on your decision. Avoid distractions.
- Organize your plan and delegate it to your team to execute as much of it as possible.
- When the situation on the ground changes or new information becomes available adapt the plan as necessary.

## DISCLOSURE

The author has no financial interests related to this article to disclose.

## REFERENCES


1. Pink DH. *A whole new mind*. Riverhead books. New York: Penguin Random House; 2005.
2. Deming WE. The essential deming: leadership principles from the father of quality. New York: McGraw Hill-Ascent and Blackstone Publishers; 2013.
3. Theodore Roosevelt: Theodore roosevelt: an autobiography. New York: The MacMillan Co; 1913.
4. Marden OS. Pushing to the front. CreateSpace Independent Publishing Platform (Kindle Direct Publishing); 2011. p. 608.
5. Lee B. Available at: https://www.facebook.com/BruceLee/posts/if-you-spend-too-much-time-thinking-about-a-thing-youll-never-get-it-done-make-a/10161561706595634/.
6. Jackson P, Delehanty H. Eleven rings: the soul of success. New York: Penguin Press; 2013. 368.
7. Maxwell JC. Developing the leaders around you: how to help others reach their full potential. New York: Harper Collins Leadership; 2005. 224.
8. King ML Jr, Harding V, King CS. Where *do we Go from here: chaos or community?* Boston, MA: Beacon Press; 2010. 256.
9. Souba WW, Souba MH. Leaders as distinction generators. Open J Leader 2018;7(2).
10. Meggison LC. Lessons from Europe for American business. SW Soc Sci Q 1963;44(1):4.
11. Ben Stein. (n.d.). AZQuotes.com. from AZQuotes.com Web site: Available at: https://www.azquotes.com/quote/282120. Accessed March 31, 2026.
12. Warren G. Bennis. (n.d.). AZQuotes.com. from AZ-Quotes.com Web site: Available at: https://www.azquotes.com/quote/1345207. Accessed March 31, 2026.
13. Michael Porter Quotes. (n.d.). BrainyQuote.com. from BrainyQuote.com Web site: Available at: https://www.brainyquote.com/quotes/michael_porter_379016. Accessed March 30, 2026.

# The Trodden and Untrodden Path

## Mentorship, Innovation, and Leadership in Dermatology

M. Hunter Bohman, DO[a,*], Brooke Bartley, MD[a], Darrell S. Rigel, MD, MS[a,b,c]

**KEYWORDS**

- Leadership • Dermatology • Mentorship • Medical education • Organized dermatology • Physician leadership • Branding

**KEY POINTS**

- Dermatology leadership develops through trodden and untrodden paths, shaped by mentorship, training, service, expertise, and creating solutions for unmet needs.
- Mentorship gives young physicians more than advice; it provides a standard for how to work, contribute, and advance through their careers with purpose.
- Credibility precedes influence. In dermatology, leadership is earned by developing real expertise, sharing knowledge generously, and becoming trusted before seeking formal titles.
- Volunteer leadership requires different skills than corporate leadership, including consensus-building, respectful persuasion, listening, and openess to change.
- Leadership is most meaningful when it prepares others to lead thorugh mentorship, education, platform-building, and shared oppurtunity.

## INTRODUCTION

Leadership is easy to describe in broad terms, but harder to see as it is being formed. By the time it appears as a presidency, invited lecturer, or national platform, much of the real work has already happened. It often begins more quietly: a mentor telling a young physician to do the work well before worrying about where it will lead, the willingness to accept an assignment when no one is watching, or the patience to listen carefully enough to realize that a practical problem deserves a new solution.

As one of Dr Rigel's fellows, I have had the privilege of seeing these lessons not only through his curriculum vitae, but in the way he works, listens, and makes room for others to grow. His lessons are rarely presented as formal lectures on leadership. They come through smaller and more memorable instructions: find your niche, do good work, take opportunities seriously, listen before deciding, and share what you learn.

This article presents both the trodden and untrodden path toward becoming a leader. The trodden path is the established one: mentorship, training, service, and expertise. The untrodden path begins when those foundations allow a physician to recognize what still needs to be built. Dr Rigel's career offers a way to understand both.

[a] Department of Dermatology, University of Texas Southwestern Medical Center, Dallas, TX 75235, USA; [b] NYU Grossman School of Medicine; [c] Cooper Clinic
* Corresponding author. Department of Dermatology, University of Texas Southwestern Medical Center, 5939 Harry Hines Boulevard, 4th Floor, Suite 100, Dallas, TX 75390.
*E-mail address:* Matthew.Bohman@utsouth-western.com

Dermatol Clin 44 (2026) 613–617
https://doi.org/10.1016/j.det.2026.06.007

## THE TRODDEN PATH BEGINS WITH MENTORSHIP

Early in his dermatology training, Dr Rigel's direction was shaped by mentors. Alfred W. Kopf, MD, was central to that development. Dr Kopf did more than introduce him to a specialty. He gave him a standard by which to build a successful and respected career.

One of the lessons Dr Rigel carried forward from that mentorship was simple: "do good work." The phrase is modest, but it contains much of what early mentorship is meant to teach. Good work means preparation, reliability, intellectual honesty, and respect for the field. It means learning the details before seeking visibility. It means becoming useful before becoming known.

This is what mentorship offers at its best. It helps a physician understand what matters before experience has fully taught the lesson. It shapes not only what one studies, but how one approaches patients, colleagues, opportunities, and responsibility. The mentorship that he received from Dr Kopf did not simply point him toward a field. It gave him a model for how to move through that field with purpose.

Having an impactful mentor is the necessary beginning. Before a physician can build something new, he or she must first learn how to walk the existing path with discipline, humility, and purpose.

## SAYING YES, SHOWING UP, AND LEARNING THE SYSTEM

The next phase of the trodden path is service.

Service is working within professional dermatology beyond the clinical setting: participating in societies, committees, educational meetings, advocacy efforts, and other efforts that help shape the specialty. The success of these organizations depends on physicians who are willing to show up, accept responsibility, and do work that may not be rewarded immediately (or ever). The key for success here is early involvement: take opportunities that become available and take them seriously, work hard, and let people view your track record over time.

The efforts leading to leadership in professional societies is cumulative. People remember who came prepared, respected others' time, followed through, treated others well, and could be trusted with a larger project the next time. Something as simple as punctuality is an important part of that standard. Being on time is one of the basic ways a physician shows respect for colleagues, trainees, patients, and the work itself. A career in this kind of service is not built in one election, lecture, or committee assignment. It is built through repeated acts of reliability. If one applies these principles, by *doing good work*, recognition from your peers will eventually ensue.

In Dr Rigel's career, that cumulative work with local and regional societies later became visible in formal leadership roles, including President of the American Academy of Dermatology (AAD), the American Society for Dermatologic Surgery, and the American Dermatologic Association, and as a Director of the American Board of Dermatology. Formal leadership positions reflect the trust of colleagues accumulated over years of preparation, follow-through, and service to the specialty.

Early on, saying yes matters. It exposes a physician to how organizations work and teaches the difference between a good idea and an executable plan. It also shows that these institutions are built by people volunteering time they could have spent elsewhere. That environment strengthens the interpersonal judgment, problem-solving, and follow-through that leadership later requires.

But saying yes should not mean saying yes on everything or forever. If being asked to do something that has little potential for positive impact on your colleagues and the specialty, save your energy for more meaningful efforts. As responsibilities grow, focus becomes necessary. A leader has to learn which opportunities fit the mission, which should be delegated, and which should be declined. Early breadth helps build perspective. Later focus helps preserve purpose.

There is also a personal side (and also potential monetary and emotional costs) that should not be ignored. Developing leadership skills requires time, travel, preparation, and often sacrifice from more people than the leader alone. Family support is critical to success as role responsibilities sometimes lead to missed family opportunities and events.

## BECOME A PROBLEM SOLVER

Leaders solve problems. They do not create them.

In Malcolm Gladwell's book, *The Tipping Point*, he describes some people as *Connectors*.[1] These are specific types of people who have the contacts, knowledge, and social skills to be effective problem solvers. The first step in being a successful problem solver is to have a network that one can reach out to, to help with a solution. So early in a career, networking is a critical step in leadership development.

To be viewed as an effective problem solver, it is not enough to solve problems—you also need to demonstrate a consistent approach that others can see and trust. You need to develop a reputation as an effective problem solver to be viewed as an effective leader. Effectiveness and trust are key for problem solving to complement leadership.

## CREDIBILITY COMES BEFORE INFLUENCE

In medicine, leadership cannot simply be claimed. It has to be earned.

The scope of Dermatology is now too broad for one to be an expert in all aspects of the field. One of Dr Rigel's recurring pieces of advice to young dermatologists is to find a niche within the specialty. A niche is not simply a branding exercise. Rather, it takes hard work and a focused plan to build real expertise, become known for doing that work well, and then sharing what you know. The niche may be clinical, research-based, educational, organizational, or advocacy-focused. The specific area matters less than the seriousness with which it is developed and the recognition that is subsequently earned.

The first goal, especially for residents and fellows, should not be to collect titles. It should be to become good enough at something that others trust you with more responsibility. Expertise leads to leadership opportunities when it is shared. A dermatologist who learns deeply and teaches generously begins to move from individual accomplishment to service. At that point, knowledge becomes useful beyond the person who holds it.

## COMMUNICATION: TURNING EXPERTISE INTO EDUCATION

Expertise does not become leadership until it can be shared.

One phrase Dr Rigel has used captures it well: "Communicators take something complicated and make it simple."[2] This quote matters here because it describes the next stage of his career. His work in melanoma and skin cancer did not remain confined to publications, lectures, or personal expertise. It became a focus on developing simple straightforward way to teach colleagues and the public to lower morbidity and mortality from that cancer. The co-development with Dr Kopf and Dr Robert Friedman of the ABCDs of early melanoma and the concept of skin self-examination represent concrete examples of this approach.

Effective preparation itself is a critical part of an effective message. A clear lecture, a well-timed presentation, and an organized argument are all key components of success. It is one way a leader makes complex information easier to receive, remember, and use.

For Dr Rigel, communication became more than presentation. It became a form of service. The practical question was not only, "What do I know?" but also, "What do other dermatologists need to know, and how can that be made useful to them to help make them better clinicians?"

That question sets up the untrodden path. Once a physician begins thinking seriously about how knowledge reaches clinicians, it becomes easier to see where existing educational structures fall short. The move from lecturer to builder, and from communication to leadership, begins there.

## UTILIZE YOUR SPECIAL SKILLS

Dermatology residency remains the most competitive field to match into. This leads to many dermatologists having impactful skill sets beyond medicine alone. Using those unique skills to differentiate someone from the *pack* can accelerate the leadership development track.

Having computer science and MBA degrees from MIT, Dr Rigel leveraged knowledge from both of those spaces to help develop and subsequently lead American Academy of Dermatology initiatives in those spaces. Beyond helping in the development of the AAD's computer office system, he helped establish the investment system and policies for the AAD's endowment funds and subsequently served 6 years as an AAD Secretary/Treasurer. This serves as an example of how recognition of hard work with excellent results leads to recognition of leadership abilities and provides an impetus toward future advancement.

## LEADERSHIP WITHOUT COMMAND

Leadership in a volunteer organization is different from leadership in a corporation.

In a professional society, expertise may open the door, but it does not guarantee followership. Much of the work depends on people who are volunteering their time because they believe in the mission, value the organization, respect the leader, or feel that their effort matters. Authority in that setting is less about command and more about trust.

This is a key distinction when discussing leadership in organized dermatology. A leader has to be willing to show people a path while remaining open to the possibility that the path may need to change. That balance is harder than it sounds. It requires conviction without stubbornness and openness without drifting.

Dr Rigel uses the quote, "Good leaders encourage followers to tell them what they need to know, not what they want to hear."[2] In Dermatology, that applies to both individuals and organizations. A leader who stops listening may mistake agreement for trust. An organization that stops listening may mistake membership for support and engagement.

Listening, however, does not mean that you must fully agree with all suggestions and requests.

One lesson Dr Rigel learned while a resident from Rudolph L. Baer, MD, then chair of dermatology at New York University, illustrates this balance. When a request was made to him that he did not want to or was unable to approve, Dr Baer listened to the request, acknowledged the reasoning behind it, and then explained clearly why the proposed solution could not work. It demonstrated another key leadership trait—that people can accept disagreement when they believe they have been heard and when the reasoning is clear.

And knowledge of what not to do is equally important in leadership development. Throughout a career, one is exposed to policies and behaviors that are clearly inappropriate. Learning how to avoid these actions during a career evolution is critical for successful leadership development.

This is also where 360-degree leadership becomes useful. As presented in Dr Rigel's 2012 AAD Clarence Livingood Plenary Lecture, this framework includes leading *up*, leading *across*, and leading *down*.[3] To be a successful leader, one must learn to respectfully influence senior leaders, collaborate with peers, and guide those being trained or supervised. In each direction, the approach is slightly different, but the principle is the same: leadership in a professional organization depends less on ordering an action than on being trusted.

## FINDING THE GAP

The untrodden path begins when a leader sees a gap that matters and is willing to build something useful in response.

For Dr Rigel, one of those gaps was access to clinically relevant practical dermatology education. Along with Mark Lebwohl, MD, and James Del Rosso, DO, he helped found the Fall Clinical Dermatology Conference more than 2 decades ago.[4] They were able to recognize a need, gather the right collaborators, and create a structure to serve the specialty.

The need was practical. Dermatologists wanted education that was current, clinically relevant, interactive, and closely tied to patient care. The conference was designed to provide *pearls of knowledge for daily use* and to maximize interaction between faculty and attendees.[5] The goal was not simply to provide more education. It was to make education practical and easier to integrate into the patient care setting.

A single lecture can transmit information, and a single meeting can bring people together. A platform has to do something more difficult: earn clinicians' attention repeatedly, adapt as the field changes, and maintain a clear identity over time.

Recognizing opportunity and developing innovative solutions is an important aspect of leadership. Building on the success of Fall Clinical, the group recognized the need for targeted education to sub-groups of the specialty and with that built a platform for over 15 subspecialty conferences. Effective leadership needs to be agile and able to respond to rapidly changing environments. When COVID hit in 2020, within 5 days the team pivoted to virtual meetings which ended up growing a whole new segment of educational offerings.

The business side of such a platform is not separate from the educational mission and also requires leadership expertise. Scheduling, faculty selection, audience engagement, financial sustainability, partnerships, and consistency all determine whether a useful idea survives beyond its first version. Without that structure, even good educational ideas can disappear. With it and strong insightful leadership, a platform can become a recurring space where clinicians learn, reconnect, and return to practice with something useable.

That is why platform-building belongs in a discussion of leadership. It requires vision, but also execution. It requires collaboration but also focus. It requires enough humility to keep asking what the audience needs and enough discipline to keep improving the format–integrating all of the attributes of effective leadership listed above. In that sense, the untrodden path is not simply the creation of something new. It is the repeated work of making that creation useful enough for others to keep walking it.

Development of this platform is not listed here simply as a career accomplishment. It is an example of leadership by construction: seeing where the existing system is incomplete, building with others, and creating a structure that allows people to learn, gather, and practice better.

## MENTORSHIP AS LEGACY

In academic medicine, mentorship is one of the few ways leadership can outlast a single career. A lecture ends. A presidency ends. A conference changes over time. But a trainee carries forward habits of thinking, standards of work, and a sense of responsibility to the field.

As Dr Rigel's fellow, I have had the opportunity to see this part of his leadership closely. He does not simply tell trainees to succeed. He pushes them to find an area where they can contribute, expects them to teach, and makes clear that leadership is not something to be claimed before it is earned. His prior fellows have gone on to build strong and meaningful careers in dermatology, integrating the approaches listed in this article and carrying forward not only his teaching but also his standard for contribution.

The best mentors do not produce copies of themselves. They produce physicians who can think, decide, communicate, and lead in their own way. Therefore, leadership development must be more than occasional advice. It requires mentoring, networking, education, real responsibility, communication skills, exposure to how organizations work, and long-term follow-up.[3]

The path therefore comes full circle. Dr Rigel was shaped by his mentors to be a leader, built his own career through expertise, helping others and organizational service, helped create new educational pathways, and now sends others forward on a path to successful careers. The measure of leadership is not only what is built, but how the next generation is effectively developed to build those that will follow them.

## SUMMARY

The trodden and untrodden paths are not competing ideas. In Dr Rigel's career, one made the other possible.

The trodden path gave him the foundation: mentorship, discipline, expertise, service, and respect for the institutions that shape the specialty. The untrodden path asked what still needed to be built. It began with the recognition that leadership is not only holding a role within existing structures, but also seeing where those structures are incomplete and helping create something useful in response.

That is what makes his career a valuable model for dermatology leadership and branding. He was shaped by mentors, then spent much of his career turning that same pattern outward: teaching, building, listening, and making room for others to grow. For those of us still early on the path, the lesson is clear enough: do good work, find the need, bring others with you, and leave the path wider than you found it.

## CLINICS CARE POINTS

- Seek mentorship early, but do not treat mentorship as passive advice. The best mentorship gives trainees standards for preparation, reliability, judgment, and contribution.
- Build credibility before seeking visibility. Choose a clinical, educational, research, advocacy, or organizational niche and develop it seriously enough that others trust your contribution.
- Say yes early to meaningful opportunities in professional societies, committees, education, and advocacy, but learn to narrow commitments as responsibilities grow.
- In volunteer leadership, persuasion matters more than command. Listen before deciding, explain disagreement clearly, and remain open to changing course when others raise valid concerns.
- Educational innovation should begin with a real unmet need. A course, meeting, platform, or brand has value only if it makes knowledge more useful to the clinicians it serves.
- Measure leadership not only by positions held, but by whether others are better prepared to lead after your involvement.

## DISCLOSURES

M.H. Bohman reports no commercial or financial conflicts of interest and no funding sources to disclose. B. Bartley reports no commercial or financial conflicts of interest and no funding sources to disclose. D.S. Rigel reports no relevant commercial or financial conflicts of interest and no funding sources to disclose. No external funding was received for this work.

## REFERENCES

1. Gladwell M. The tipping point: how little things can make a big difference. Boston: Little, Brown and Company; 2000.
2. Rigel DS. Presidential address. Presented at: american dermatological Association annual meeting; 2007. Unpublished lecture slides. Used with permission.
3. Rigel DS. Influencing the Direction of Our Specialty: How an Effective Organization Can Make a Difference. Clarence Livingood Lecture. Presented at: American Academy of Dermatology Annual Meeting; March 18, 2012; San Diego, CA. Unpublished lecture slides. Used with permission.
4. Buchanan L. What to expect at the 2023 fall clinical dermatology conference. Dermatology times. 2023. Available at: https://www.dermatologytimes.com/view/what-to-expect-at-the-2023-fall-clinical-dermatology-conference. Accessed June 3, 2026.
5. Winter clinical dermatology shines in Hawaii. The dermatologist. 2016. Available at: www.hmpgloballearningnetwork.com/site/thederm/site/cathlab/event/winter-clinical-dermatology-shines-hawaii. Accessed June 3, 2026.

# Effective Organizational Leadership

Seemal R. Desai, MD[a,b,*]

**KEYWORDS**

• Leadership • Organizational leadership • Dermatology • Conflict management • Political savvy • Medical societies • Strategic planning • Professional development

**KEY POINTS**

- Effective organizational leaders unite constituencies by listening first, soliciting all perspectives, and deferring personal opinions until the voices of all stakeholders have been heard.
- Proactive conflict anticipation allows identification of tensions before they escalate and is a defining hallmark of high-performing leaders in medical organizations.
- Meticulous documentation and transparent record-keeping build institutional trust, protect the organization during disputes, and provide a roadmap for successors.
- Political savviness combined with diplomatic communication allows leaders to advance organizational priorities while preserving relationships and maintaining credibility.
- Thinking ahead while envisioning the long arc of organizational needs is what distinguishes transactional managers from transformational leaders.

## INTRODUCTION

Dermatologists are trained to diagnose, treat, and advocate for patients. Increasingly, however, the specialty demands leaders who can also guide complex organizations—medical societies, academic departments, private practices, hospital systems, regulatory bodies, and advocacy coalitions. The leap from clinician to organizational leader is not automatic. It requires the deliberate cultivation of a different kind of intelligence: one that is relational, strategic, emotionally disciplined, and forward-looking.

The author has spent the better part of 2 decades navigating the full continuum of organized dermatology, ranging from roles such as serving as President of the Dallas/Fort Worth Dermatological Society, to leading the Texas Dermatological Society, to serving as President of the Skin of Color Society, to being elected to the Board of Directors of the American Academy of Dermatology (AAD), and ultimately to serving as President of the AAD—the world's largest dermatologic society—as its youngest ever elected president. Each of these roles has deepened the understanding of what it truly means to lead an organization effectively.

This article distills those lessons into a practical framework for organizational leadership: how to unite diverse constituencies, how to lead by listening, how to anticipate conflicts before they erupt, how to maintain the records and documentation that protect the organization, and how to navigate the political landscape of organized medicine with diplomacy and integrity.

## DEFINING ORGANIZATIONAL LEADERSHIP IN MEDICINE

Leadership theory has evolved considerably over the past several decades. Transactional leadership—based on the exchange of rewards for performance—has largely given way to transformational leadership models, which focus on

[a] Innovative Dermatology, Dallas, TX, USA; [b] Department of Dermatology, University of Texas Southwestern Medical Center, Dallas, TX, USA
* Department of Dermatology, University of Texas Southwestern Medical Center, Dallas, TX.
*E-mail address:* seemald@yahoo.com

Dermatol Clin 44 (2026) 619–624
https://doi.org/10.1016/j.det.2026.06.008

| Abbreviation | |
|---|---|
| AAD | American Academy of Dermatology |

inspiring and motivating followers toward a higher collective vision.[1] In medical organizations, transformational leadership is particularly relevant because the leader's followers are often peers: accomplished, independent-minded clinicians who are not compelled by hierarchy alone.

Kouzes and Posner, in their foundational work The Leadership Challenge, identified 5 practices of exemplary leaders: modeling the way, inspiring a shared vision, challenging the process, enabling others to act, and encouraging the heart.[2] Each of these practices translates directly to the medical society context, where the leader must be part-diplomat, part-strategist, and part-servant.

Within dermatology specifically, organizational leaders must contend with a unique ecosystem: membership bodies with diverse political viewpoints, subspecialty tensions, generational divides, private practice versus academic fissures, and the ever-present pressure of regulatory and legislative change. The effective leader must hold all of these dynamics simultaneously while keeping the organization focused on its mission.

## THE UNITING IMPERATIVE: LEADING WITH UNITY

Perhaps the most foundational principle of effective organizational leadership is the commitment to unity. An organization fractured along ideological, subspecialty, or political lines cannot execute its mission. The leader's first obligation is to bring people together, not by suppressing difference, but by creating structures and cultures in which difference is honored and channeled productively.

Unity does not mean unanimity. It means establishing a shared sense of purpose that transcends individual disagreements. In practical terms, this requires the leader to be deliberate about inclusion from the outset of their tenure. Every significant decision should be preceded by a process of broad consultation. Stakeholders who are rarely heard must be actively sought out. Minority viewpoints must be given oxygen even when the majority has already formed a consensus.

Research on inclusive leadership supports this approach. A study published in *Harvard Business Review* found that teams with inclusive leaders were 17% more likely to report high performance, 20% more likely to report high decision-making quality, and 29% more likely to report collaborative behavior.[3] These findings are directly applicable to volunteer-led medical organizations, where engagement and buy-in cannot be assumed.

## THE DISCIPLINE OF LISTENING: WITHHOLDING OPINION UNTIL ALL VOICES ARE HEARD

One of the most counterintuitive and powerful disciplines of effective leadership is knowing when not to speak. Leaders, by virtue of their position and experience, often carry strong opinions into deliberations. When those opinions are expressed early, they tend to close down conversation: other participants defer to the leader's view, dissenting voices go quiet, and the richness of collective wisdom is squandered.

Active listening which is defined as the full concentration on, understanding of, and response to a speaker, is widely recognized in the organizational behavior literature as a foundational leadership competency.[4] But truly effective leaders practice something even more disciplined: they withhold their own opinions until the room has had its full say. This deliberate reticence signals respect for all participants, prevents premature closure, and often surfaces considerations the leader would not have generated independently.

The author has consistently practiced this principle across every leadership role: arriving at governance meetings with a clear understanding of the agenda but without predetermined positions; asking open-ended questions rather than leading questions; allowing silence after a question, resisting the urge to fill it; and responding to contributions with synthesis rather than judgment. Over time, this approach builds a culture in which members feel safe to speak candidly, which is the precondition for the kind of honest deliberation organizations need to make sound decisions.

Stephen Covey articulated this principle elegantly: seek first to understand, then to be understood.[5] In the organizational leadership context, this is not merely a communication tactic—it is a moral stance. It says: your voice matters. Your perspective is worth my full attention before I offer my own.

## PROACTIVE CONFLICT MANAGEMENT: ANTICIPATING TENSIONS BEFORE THEY ARISE

Conflict is inevitable in any organization composed of passionate, high-achieving individuals. What distinguishes effective leaders is not their ability to resolve conflicts after they erupt, but their ability to anticipate tensions before they reach crisis proportions.

Proactive conflict management begins with environmental scanning: the systematic attention to undercurrents, alliances, grievances, and historical patterns within the organization. New leaders should invest heavily in understanding the organizational memory, what conflicts have occurred in the past, how they were resolved (or not), and what residual tensions remain. This intelligence, gathered through one-on-one conversations, committee minutes, and informal channels, is invaluable.

Thomas and Kilmann's conflict mode instrument identifies five approaches to conflict: competing, collaborating, compromising, avoiding, and accommodating.[6] Effective organizational leaders do not default to any single mode; they deploy different approaches based on the nature and stakes of the conflict. However, at the organizational level, prevention is the superordinate strategy. A leader who identifies a brewing tension between 2 committee chairs and convenes a private, facilitated conversation before the tension becomes public has done more for organizational health than any amount of post-hoc mediation.

In practice, proactive conflict management involves several habits. First, maintaining a pulse on the organization's emotional climate through regular informal check-ins with key stakeholders. Second, identifying issues that have the potential to divide the membership, examples including legislative positions, dues structures, scope-of-practice policies, and designing deliberative processes that build consensus before positions are finalized. Third, creating explicit channels for dissent so that frustrations are aired in constructive forums rather than in hallways or social media.

## DOCUMENTATION AND RECORD-KEEPING: THE ARCHITECTURE OF ORGANIZATIONAL INTEGRITY

In the day-to-day urgency of organizational leadership, documentation can feel like an administrative afterthought. In fact, it is one of the most consequential habits a leader can cultivate. Meticulous records protect the organization legally, ensure continuity of institutional memory, facilitate accountability, and provide the foundation for evidence-based decision-making.

Documentation in organizational leadership encompasses several distinct domains: minutes of governance meetings; records of decisions made and the rationale behind them; communications with external stakeholders, regulatory bodies, and government agencies; financial records; and the documentation of conflicts of interest and their management. Each of these record types serves a different protective function, but all share a common attribute: they create a factual record that cannot be rewritten retroactively.

The importance of documentation is amplified in medical societies and professional organizations, where decisions can affect thousands of members, influence regulatory policy, and carry significant financial implications. In this environment, a leader who is scrupulous about documentation not only protects the organization but also demonstrates to the membership that governance is transparent and accountable.

Equally important is the documentation of process, and not just of outcomes. When a contested decision is made, a record of how that decision was reached (who was consulted, what alternatives were considered, what dissenting views were expressed) is as valuable as the decision itself. If the decision is later challenged, the process record demonstrates that it was made in good faith, with appropriate deliberation.

## POLITICAL SAVVINESS AND DIPLOMATIC LEADERSHIP

The phrase "playing politics" carries negative connotations in most professional cultures, suggesting manipulation, self-interest, and backroom dealing. But political savviness—properly understood—is a legitimate and essential leadership competency. It refers to the ability to understand the informal power structures, influence networks, and unspoken rules of an organization, and to navigate them in service of the organization's mission rather than personal advancement.

Ferris and colleagues defined political skill as a multidimensional construct encompassing social astuteness, interpersonal influence, networking ability, and apparent sincerity.[7] High political skill, they found, is associated with greater leadership effectiveness, career success, and the ability to manage stressful situations. Crucially, *apparent sincerity* with being perceived as genuine and non-manipulative is a component of political skill, not its antithesis. The most politically skilled leaders are not those who are most calculating, rather they are those who have internalized their values so thoroughly that their navigation of complex social terrain truly is authentic.

In the context of organized medicine, political savviness involves understanding which stakeholders have formal authority and which have informal influence; knowing when to advocate publicly and when to work quietly behind the scenes; reading the room before making a motion; building coalitions before a vote rather than lobbying after one fails; and knowing when to push and when to wait. It is the practical intelligence of a leader who understands that even the best ideas require strategic implementation to succeed.

Diplomatic leadership complements political savviness by providing the communication framework. Diplomacy in leadership means delivering difficult messages with care, disagreeing without disrespecting, maintaining relationships with those whose positions you have opposed, and finding language that acknowledges competing interests while articulating a path forward. The skilled diplomatic leader can say "no" to a proposal without saying "no" to the person who proposed it.

One of the most powerful diplomatic tools available to organizational leaders is the individual private conversation. Before a contentious vote, before a public statement, before major announcements, the leader who has taken the time to speak individually with key stakeholders has already done the most important political work. Surprises erode trust, and, conversely, advance consultation and dialogue builds it.

## THINKING AHEAD: LEADING FROM THE STRATEGIC HORIZON

Effective organizational leaders do not just manage the present, rather they actively shape the future. This forward-looking orientation, often called strategic thinking, is what distinguishes transformational leaders from transactional administrators. Strategic leaders ask not only "What does the organization need today?" but "What will the organization need in three years, five years, ten years, and how do we begin preparing for it now?"

In medical professional societies, strategic thinking requires actively monitoring the external environment, and translating these signals into organizational priorities. In dermatology, this can include legislative changes, workforce trends, technological disruption, demographic shifts in the patient population and the physician workforce. It also requires attention to the internal landscape: the health of the leadership pipeline, the financial sustainability of programs, and the relevance of the organization's offerings to the next generation of members.

The concept of *horizon scanning*, which is the systematic identification of emerging issues that may affect the organization in the medium to long term, has been increasingly applied in health care governance.[8] Leaders who practice horizon scanning are not caught off guard by predictable changes; they have already begun the strategic conversation about how the organization will respond.

Thinking ahead also applies at the interpersonal and political level. Before taking a position, the effective leader considers not just the immediate consequences but the downstream effects: How will this position be perceived by different segments of the membership? What precedent does it set? What relationships might it strain or strengthen? How will it look in 2 years if the landscape has changed? This kind of anticipatory thinking does not produce paralysis—it produces better, more durable decisions.

## LEADERSHIP STYLE IN CONTEXT: ADAPTING TO THE ORGANIZATION

No single leadership style is universally effective. The most sophisticated leaders are stylistically flexible, adapting their approach to the needs of the situation. Situational leadership theory, developed by Hersey and Blanchard, proposes that the appropriate leadership style depends on the readiness level of the followers and the nature of the task.[9] A newly formed committee with little experience needs more directive guidance; a mature committee of seasoned professionals needs facilitation, not direction.

In the context of large medical organizations, the most effective overarching style is servant leadership, which truly means the orientation toward the growth and well-being of the people and communities one serves.[10–15] Servant leaders place the needs of the organization and its members above their own advancement. They measure their success not by the recognition they receive but by the legacy they leave: a stronger organization, a deeper leadership pipeline, a culture of inclusion and excellence.

This orientation is not passive. Servant leaders are often among the most decisive and directionally clear individuals in an organization. The distinction is motivational: they are pursuing institutional good, not personal aggrandizement. When a servant leader makes a hard decision such as cuts a program, terminates a partnership, takes an unpopular legislative position, the membership may disagree, but they rarely question the leader's intentions.

The author's own leadership style has been shaped by these principles: lead by listening, unite before deciding, anticipate before reacting, document everything, be politically savvy without being manipulative, and always thinking about what comes next, not just what is in front of you.

## BUILDING THE NEXT GENERATION OF LEADERS

A leader's most enduring legacy is the leaders they develop. No organization can sustain excellence without a robust pipeline of emerging leaders who are ready, willing, and equipped to serve. This requires intentional investment: creating mentorship structures, designing entry-level governance opportunities, offering leadership development education, and identifying and encouraging individuals who might not self-nominate without prompting.

Diversity in the leadership pipeline is not merely a social good, rather it is an organizational imperative. Organizations whose leadership reflects the diversity of their membership make better decisions, represent their constituencies more accurately, and are more resilient in the face of change. Leaders who have occupied positions of privilege have a particular responsibility to use their platform to open doors for those who have historically been excluded.

The author, as chair of the AAD's Leadership Development Steering Committee and as AAD President, made the cultivation of early career leaders a central priority, because an organization that does not invest in its next generation is borrowing against its own future. Effective mentorship means more than encouragement; it means providing concrete sponsorship, creating opportunities for visibility, and advocating for emerging leaders when they are not in the room.

## THE GOVERNANCE–STAFF RELATIONSHIP

In large professional societies, the relationship between elected governance (board members, officers) and professional staff (executive directors, staff attorneys, policy analysts) is a perennial source of tension. Governance leaders who micromanage staff undermine expertise and morale; those who defer too completely abdicate their fiduciary responsibility. Effective leaders invest time in establishing clear role boundaries, building trusting relationships with senior staff, and creating governance structures that enable strategic oversight without operational intrusion.

## SOCIAL MEDIA AND ORGANIZATIONAL VOICE

The proliferation of social media has created new pressures on organizational leaders. Individual leaders now have platforms that can reach thousands of members and non-members instantly. This creates both opportunity and risk. Personal social media activity by organizational leaders can be misread as official organizational positions, can inflame rather than resolve conflicts, and can create reputational hazards. Effective leaders are deliberate about distinguishing their personal voice from their institutional role, and they model the kind of civil discourse they wish to see in the broader professional community.

## MANAGING GOVERNANCE IN AN ERA OF POLITICAL POLARIZATION

Medical professional societies operate in an increasingly polarized political environment, in which even seemingly clinical questions can become politically freighted. Leaders who are perceived as politically partisan in either direction lose the ability to represent the full breadth of their membership. Navigating this terrain requires a disciplined commitment to leading with evidence, framing positions in terms of patient welfare and professional integrity, and resisting the temptation to align the organization with partisan political movements even when doing so might seem expedient.

## SUMMARY

Effective organizational leadership in dermatology is a learnable, practicable skill set, not a fixed trait reserved for a select few. It demands the discipline to listen before speaking, the foresight to anticipate conflicts before they erupt, the rigor to document everything that matters, the savviness to navigate the informal power landscape without compromising one's integrity, and the vision to lead not just for today but for the organization's future.

These principles are not abstract ideals. They are habits of mind and practice that can be cultivated deliberately, refined through experience, and transmitted to the next generation of leaders. The dermatology community has a rich tradition of physician-leaders who have shaped not only the specialty but the broader landscape of American medicine. That tradition will be sustained by those who lead with authenticity, humility, and an unwavering commitment to the collective good.

## CLINICS CARE POINTS

- Lead by listening: withhold your opinion in deliberative settings until every stakeholder has been heard. This practice prevents premature closure and builds the trust that makes decisive action possible.
- Anticipate conflict proactively: scan the organizational environment regularly for emerging tensions and address them through

facilitated dialogue before they reach governance bodies.

- Document rigorously: maintain decision logs, meeting minutes, and process records that capture not just what was decided but how and why. This protects the organization and establishes accountability.
- Practice diplomatic political savviness: understand informal power structures and use that knowledge in service of the organization's mission, not personal advancement. Test your actions against the transparency standard: would you be comfortable if the full membership could see exactly what you are doing and why?
- Think across time horizons: the best organizational leaders are simultaneously managing today's agenda and preparing for tomorrow's challenges. Invest in horizon scanning, succession planning, and leadership pipeline development.
- Model servant leadership: measure your effectiveness not by the recognition you receive but by the strength of the organization and the depth of the leadership bench you leave behind.

## FUNDING

None.

## DISCLOSURES

The author discloses that he has served as a leader of multiple dermatologic and non-dermatologic organizations and currently serves as President of the Global Vitiligo Foundation.

## REFERENCES

1. Bass BM, Riggio RE. Transformational leadership. 2nd edition. Mahwah (NJ): Lawrence Erlbaum Associates; 2006.
2. Kouzes JM, Posner BZ. The leadership challenge: how to make extraordinary things happen in organizations. 6th edition. Hoboken (NJ): Wiley; 2017.
3. Bourke J, Dillon B. The diversity and inclusion revolution: eight powerful truths. Deloitte Review 2018; 22:82–95.
4. Rogers CR, Farson RE. Active listening. In: Newman RG, Danzinger MA, Cohen M, editors. Communicating in business today. Washington DC: Heath and Company; 1987.
5. Covey SR. The 7 habits of highly effective people: restoring the character ethic. New York: Free Press; 1989.
6. Thomas KW, Kilmann RH. Thomas-Kilmann conflict mode instrument. Mountain View (CA): Xicom; 1974.
7. Ferris GR, Treadway DC, Perrewé PL, et al. Political skill in organizations. J Manag 2007;33(3):290–320.
8. Foresight Horizon Scanning Centre. Scenario planning. London: Government Office for Science; 2009.
9. Hersey P, Blanchard KH. Management of organizational behavior: utilizing human resources. 4th edition. Englewood Cliffs (NJ): Prentice-Hall; 1982.
10. Greenleaf RK. Servant leadership: a journey into the nature of legitimate power and greatness. New York: Paulist Press; 1977.
11. Desai SR. Assumes presidency of the American Academy of Dermatology. AAD News Release 2024. Available at: https://www.aad.org/news/seemal-desai-new-president-aad.
12. Desai S. Leadership in dermatology. Orlando (FL): Presented at: Skin of Color Society Scientific Symposium; 2025.
13. Edmondson AC. The fearless Organization: creating psychological safety in the workplace for learning, innovation, and growth. Hoboken (NJ): Wiley; 2018.
14. Goleman D. Leadership that gets results. Harv Bus Rev 2000;78(2):78–90.
15. Collins J. Good to great: why some companies make the leap... and others don't. New York: HarperCollins; 2001.

# Leadership by Building Your Own Personal Brand

Terrence A. Cronin Jr, MD[a,b,*], Christian MacDonald, BS[c]

**KEYWORDS**

• Dermatology • Leadership • Brand • Branding • Leader • Instagram

**KEY POINTS**

- Professional and personal success depends on the recognition of your value by others.
- Personal branding is a strategic practice to promote your value and define your leadership qualities.
- Practice branding is the visual representation of your practice to patients and the public.
- Personal branding and leadership requires work and authenticity.
- Branding enhances your credibility and promotes potential opportunities.

## BACKGROUND

In the journey toward personal and professional success, one key element is often overlooked—the power of building and developing your own brand. Personal branding is vital in today's world where everyone is essentially a brand themselves. However, personal branding is not just about how you present yourself to others: it should be a billboard promoting you on your path to leadership. In today's competitive health care landscape, building trust with patients is crucial for physicians. As medical practitioners, you not only need to provide quality health care but also establish a strong brand identity that resonates with your patients and your colleagues.[1] Doctor branding goes beyond a mere logo or slogan; it encompasses the values, expertise, and patient-centered approach that doctors bring to their practice.

Your brand is not just about how you present yourself; it is the narrative that others collectively hold about you. As Jeff Bezos rightly said, "Your brand is what people say about you when you're not in the room."[2] Your goal should be to ensure that the narrative created about you is accurate, compelling, and helpful to your mission.

## DISCUSSION

Much of your professional and personal success depends on persuading others to recognize your value. You need to do this in job applications, when seeking promotions, vying for leadership positions, or even in the dating scene. In Jill Avery and Rachel Greenwald's recent Harvard Business Review article *A new approach to building your personal brand*, they warned that "[f]or better or worse, in today's world everyone is a brand, and you need to develop yours and get comfortable marketing it."[3]

Personal branding is an intentional, strategic practice in which you define and express your own value proposition. And though people have always carefully cultivated their public personas and reputations, online search engines and social media have greatly expanded the potential audience for—and risks and rewards associated with—such efforts. For example, if your personal value proposition is to be a strong leader who is warm, empathetic, and able to deliver results, how would you exhibit and showcase these attributes?

Todd Shryock, a managing editor of *Medical Economics*, attests, "For many physicians, marketing their practice can feel like unfamiliar

[a] Frost Department of Dermatology and Cutaneous Surgery, University of Miami, University of Miami Miller School of Medicine, Miami, FL 33136, USA; [b] Cronin Skin Cancer Center, 1399 S Harbor City Boulevard, Melbourne, FL 32901, USA; [c] Florida State University College of Medicine, Tallahassee, FL, USA
* Corresponding author. Cronin Skin Cancer Center, 1399 S Harbor City Boulevard, Melbourne, FL 32901.
*E-mail address:* TCRonin2@aol.com

Dermatol Clin 44 (2026) 625–631
https://doi.org/10.1016/j.det.2026.05.005

territory. Trained to diagnose, treat, and care for patients, doctors often have little formal education in how to build a professional brand, attract new patients, or communicate their value in a crowded health care marketplace. Yet, in today's competitive environment, marketing is no longer optional—it's essential. One of the biggest challenges doctors face is balancing the business side of medicine with the clinical side. Physicians may hesitate to promote themselves out of concern that it seems self-serving or at odds with their professional image. At the same time, patients have more choices than ever, and they frequently turn to online reviews, practice websites, and social media when deciding where to seek care. A lack of visibility can leave even highly skilled physicians overlooked."[4]

When I entered the leadership track of my medical specialty, it struck me that I needed a catchphrase to inspire dermatologists and jump-start our mission. Associating that phrase with my persona meant that our members would always link me with that mission. *Stay passionate about dermatology*! was born and became the brand that I signed all my professional messages with at the American Academy of Dermatology. I even made sure my social media handle was aligned and ready with @passionfordermatology. This personal brand was a strong one and proved motivational to my colleagues.[5]

Avery and Greenwald emphasize that *a strong, well-managed personal brand benefits you in several ways. It enhances your visibility, particularly among those who matter to you and to the things you hope to accomplish. It can also help you expand your network and attract new opportunities. And on a deeper level, the process of building one can help you uncover, celebrate, and share the unique abilities you bring to the world.*[3]

To build a strong personal brand, it is essential to follow a strategic approach. Here are 10 steps[4] to help you cultivate your brand image.

1. Identify your target audience.
2. Research your competitors and industry landscape.
3. Define your brand's purpose and position.
4. Develop a consistent personality and brand voice.
5. Create a catchy catchphrase.
6. Craft your personal story to engage and resonate with others.
7. Write a memorable slogan that encapsulates your brand essence.
8. Design a visually appealing brand look and logo.
9. Integrate your brand into all aspects of your life, including social media, business, and presentations.
10. Do not be afraid to rebrand and adapt as needed to stay relevant and authentic.

By following these steps, your office can establish its own brand—one with boldness, efficiency, and the ability to encapsulate your mission to your patients. As such, each of these steps will be elaborated on, using specific examples of successful methods regarding each principle.

### Step 1: Identify Your Target Audience

While elaborating on this principle may seem trivial given the inherently assumed simplicity of the goal of branding, it is imperative that identifying your target audience is done correctly to maximize appropriate exposure to those who should see your message. For instance, hypothetically, you own and operate an obstetrics/gynecology practice. Immediately, you would most likely think that women are your target audience. However, when building your own brand, you should think bigger than that. Your target audience is all of the adults in your community since men also would inform their spouses about your practice if branded correctly. This goes to show that your target audience is not limited to your potential patients, but rather to anyone and everyone who would be inclined after exposure to your brand to inform potential patients of your quality services.

### Step 2: Research Your Competitors and Industry Landscape

Knowing the competitive terrain is important for success. An old doctor's joke touches on this idea. *What do you call a doctor in the next town*? *A colleague*. *What do you call a doctor in your own town*? *Competition*. In preparation, you should analyze the other physicians in your specialty that practice in your community. What are their strengths and weaknesses and how do they position themselves online? Perhaps you can fill gaps that they aren't focused on.[6] It is also a great idea to pay attention to how successful colleagues in other communities position themselves.

Consider offering services that aren't provided in your community like aesthetics, ultraviolet light therapy, biologics, Mohs surgery, lasers, and intense pulsed light (IPL). Avoid the pitfall of copying competitors as your authenticity is appreciated and will lead to patient retention.

### *Step 3: Define Your Brand's Purpose and Position*

This step acts as the main basis of your brand. Without this, your message can be unclear, steering your prospective audience's attention away from your services. Additionally, this step encompasses the leadership aspect of our thesis: your leadership can be exemplified through your brand's purpose and position as it illustrates your implicit values. Despite its clear importance, this can also be the most difficult step for physicians to complete. In this instance, it is best to think big and return to the basics. What do you value as a physician? What do you value as a human? What brief message can you present to an audience that would allow them to effectively understand your values?[7] Once you get past these 3 questions, the rest is downhill and the following steps will delineate various methods to present your values.

### *Step 4: Develop a Consistent Personality and Brand Voice*

Now that you have defined your brand's purpose and position, it is time to establish your brand's personality and voice. This entails contemplating the technique and style in which you present your messages.[8] Some quick questions you may ask yourself include: Do I want to present my practice more formally or informally? Do I want to focus on presenting my services given my credibility, humor to attract attention, or from a logical perspective? There are a plethora of ways to combine these thoughts, as well. If a more formal approach is decided upon, establishing credibility with the audience best accomplishes this goal; however, if a more informal approach is selected, humor could be beneficial to garner attention to your services. A good comparison for these aspects would be the contrast between a Morgan & Morgan television advertisement and a Doritos Super Bowl commercial. While both accomplish their goals for the advertisement, they go about such in stark manners. On one hand, the Morgan & Morgan advertisement focuses on their accomplishments in what financial aid they have been able to salvage from their clients' cases. On the other hand, the Doritos Super Bowl commercial often uses humor via unorthodox, comedically strewn situations and dilemmas to leave the audience laughing but also thinking about Doritos products. Thus, while both organizations employed drastically different methodologies to promote their services/products, they both accomplish their advertising goal, nonetheless. So, for your practice, having your values and message aligned is great, but how do you wish to portray these to an audience?

### *Step 5: Create a Memorable Catchphrase*

While this is a simple step, it does require a level of creativity to yield success. Nevertheless, first contemplate 3 to 5 words that encapsulate your values as a brand and medical practice. Once you have these in mind, ponder alliterations that could be used in conjunction with those words. This will give you a solid basis on which you can construct your catchphrase. Following this, present these ideas that you have created to others who understand your values. This could include your coworkers, family, or friends. Ask them which of your ideas that they favor and also inquire about their ideas on how to expand your ideas. This garners the most quality attention to your ideas whilst sparking creativity amongst likeminded individuals that understand the purpose that this catchphrase needs to serve.

### *Step 6: Craft Your Personal Story to Engage and Resonate with Others*

Storytelling has been a part of the human experience and predates recorded history. We use stories to connect with others, experience emotions, and to feel understood. In business, storytelling plays a critical role in driving change, building trust and credibility.[9] According to a study by Prezi, a web-based presentation tool provider, 55% of people say that a great story captures their focus and keeps them engaged.[10]

You need to create a story that is compelling and relevant to your practice and the concerns of your patients. Why is the information that you are sharing relevant to your patients?

The inclusion of a conflict that you worked through helps your patients stay engaged as they anticipate and try to mentally solve what the story's resolution will be. Sharing stories helps humanize the decision-making process and positions you as the shepherd to help them make the right choices.

### *Step 7: Write a Memorable Slogan that Encapsulates Your Brand Essence*

While many might argue that this step is immensely similar to Step 5, there are a few key characteristics that separate the importance of a memorable slogan from a catchy catchphrase. Mainly, the slogan provides a broader context for your practice, whereas the catchphrase is a quick, precise mode of communication to your audience. Thus, we need to generate this slogan to express the truth behind your brand essence. Similar to the process of crafting your catchphrase, think of a few words that represent your values. However, instead of thinking of creative mannerisms to present these values, think more logically and craft a sentence for each word that portrays your brand. Once again, present these sentences to your workers, family, and friends, ask for their opinions regarding these sentences, and further inquire if they thought of any ideas that would help better illustrate the brand.

### Step 8: Design a Visually Appealing Brand Look and Logo

This step most certainly requires the most creativity out of all the steps. The best recommendation would be to keep it simple. You do not want to present an overcomplicated logo to your audience.[11] Rather, select a symbol that best embodies your brand and surround it with coordinating colors. For example, in my Dermatology practice, I use a cartoon sun surrounded by yellow, green, and blue hues to present my mission. It is simple yet extremely effective at conveying what I do in my practice.

### Step 9: Integrate Your Brand into all Aspects of Your Life, including Social Media, Business, and Presentations

Now that you have garnered a solid brand from the previous steps, it is time to apply your brand to areas where you can promote yourself and your brand. The most obvious platforms to input your brand is social media, professional presentations, and in-office communications. Social media platforms speak to the public and include but are not limited to Facebook, Instagram, LinkedIn, Threads, Tik-Tok, and X (formerly Twitter). Your professional presentations can use your logo and design work to make any PowerPoint presentation memorable. In-office communications speak directly to your patient and includes practice letterhead, patient handouts, and the lobby television. It is easy to be a star in your own lobby, and you can have your television programming on rotation. I recommend using subtitles and keeping the volume off to avoid disturbing repetition. Rotating screen messages can also be used in your clinic examination rooms.

### Step 10: Do Not Be Afraid to Rebrand and Adapt as Needed to Stay Relevant and Authentic

The willingness to change demonstrates one key aspect of an open mindset in addition to promoting success. It is easier said than done, though. When your brand begins to feel stale, it is vital that you incorporate new ideas to adapt to the competitive workplace to stay relevant and authentic, but this does not need to be done at the expense of your values. Instead, consistently researching new modes of communication, design tools to enhance your logos, or what has become popular in your field allows you to be best prepared to rebrand when need be.[12] Additionally, by being open-minded with regard to rebranding, you are being proactive to ensure that your brand maintains the high level of success that your quality health care deserves.

There are now more things to consider when establishing your personal brand given the modern era. The contemporary digital landscape brings both opportunities and challenges. Search engine optimization, content creation, and online reputation management are now central to practice growth, but they require consistent attention and expertise. Digital strategies are becoming a must-have for all organizations, including physician's private practices. Physicians who are already stretched thin by clinical duties, administrative tasks, and regulatory requirements may find it difficult to devote time and resources to marketing, but a practice's digital presence is often the go-to for patients, prospective patients, those in your community, referral sources, and others who want to know more about you.

There is also the challenge of differentiation. In fields where an extended number of practices offer similar services, how can a physician stand out? Communicating a clear value proposition, highlighting patient-centered care, and fostering authentic connections are critical—but not always easy to execute without guidance. One of the primary goals of doctor branding is to establish credibility and showcase expertise. Patients want assurance that their health care provider is competent and knowledgeable. By highlighting educational qualifications, specialized training, and certifications, doctors can demonstrate their expertise. Engaging in continuous professional development and staying updated with the latest advancements in their field further enhances their credibility. Positioning yourself as a thought leader and medical authority requires dedication and involvement in your specialty. Building on your authority and sharing with the public begins with showcasing your practice, achievements, and innovative ideas on platforms such as blogs, medical journals, and physician networks. All of these allow you to demonstrate your expertise and credibility in your field.

Finally, doctors must navigate ethical boundaries. Marketing in health care must balance honesty, transparency, and professionalism with the need to attract patients. Overpromising results or using aggressive tactics can damage trust, making it all the more important for physicians to approach marketing with care.[4] Clear and effective communication is essential in doctor branding. Doctors should communicate in a language that patients understand, avoiding complex medical jargon. Actively listening to patients' concerns and questions and providing comprehensive explanations can foster trust and confidence. Engaging with patients through active dialogue and establishing a patient-doctor relationship built on trust are key elements of effective communication.

Solid branding is vital for private practice physicians to ensure they are delivering a clear consistent message about their practice.[13] The branding of your medical practice is the visual representation of your practice to patients and the outside world. It is imperative to make sure your branding is consistent in all your marketing: professional, digital, and physical outlets. Often, branding consistency can decrease to the wayside when the physician or owner decides to update aspects of the practice but decides against fully updating all the practice outlets. This may mean that new providers were added, additional locations opened, name changes, color schemes altered, or all the above. It can be a great idea to give your logo a much-needed facelift if it's dated but make sure that when you launch the new logo and colors schemes it makes its way to all aspects of the medical practice. Inconsistent logos, business cards, and colors will cause confusion and can look sloppy or cheap. An example of inconsistent branding for a medical practice could be if a doctor was recently employed at a local hospital or physicians' group but has branched out and become an independent private practice physician. The physician may have outdated business cards with the old hospital logo or colors, or the website is different from the previous employers. This will cause confusion for potential patients who might want to schedule an appointment. If they are under the impression the physician is employed by the hospital, they may be under the assumption that the practice accepts a certain insurance or that the medical records are already in the system. Patients become frustrated and confused when they discover there may be changes to their appointment. Inconsistency in your medical practice branding can reflect a lack of diligence or professionalism.

When talking about consistency for all outlets of your medical practice, what are some of the common health care marketing outlets used by doctors that could have inconsistent marketing?

- Logo
- Marketing collateral
- Social media
- Google and search platforms
- Business Listings
- Signage
- Digital Advertising
- Print & Outdoor Advertising

Branding is an opportunity for private practice physicians to market their medical practice.[13,14] Health care marketing involves networking with other health care professionals and potential patients. Your brand helps other physicians and health care professionals associate visually with your practice. You want your medical branding to be memorable, clean, consistent, and deliver a clear message. As a physician your brand is the visual way to represent your practice in business and marketing, your reputation depends on it.

Your first impression is particularly important. Branding is the frontline of your health care marketing as a physician. Invest the money and design your logo in a legible, medical friendly font with 2 to 3 colors maximum. Blues and reds are among the most patient-friendly colors in the medical industries so choosing a variation of these can be a smart decision. Once you have a logo that you are proud of then you can invest the energy in a website that will serve as the digital billboard and foundation of your digital brand. Carry these tips across social media banners, social media graphics & posts, advertising, etc. to keep everything consistent and clean.

In the digital age, a strong online presence is vital for doctor branding.[15] Using social media platforms, doctors can attract potential patients, share educational content, and establish thought leadership in their field. By maintaining a professional website, optimizing online profiles, and showcasing patient testimonials, doctors can strengthen their brand and attract new patients.

It may be helpful to seek expert guidance and education by partnering with a digital marketing consultant or taking targeted courses on personal branding and digital marketing. You can also get support from online networks where doctors exchange expertise, share experiences, and support one another in managing their professional reputations. Communicate with your consultant about how you want your brand to look and trust in their health care marketing expertise. You may be an incredible physician, and your referring doctors know that, but when looking over your marketing material do they associate your brand with your high-quality health care services?[16] Does your branding differentiate your medical practice from other doctors in your profession?

Branding says a lot about your practice and the physicians that are part of it. Be meticulous, especially early on in creating your brand, that it communicates your core values, medical approach, and overall vision. Then, once you have a brand in place that you are proud of, set up processes and procedures to ensure they are adhered to in all aspects of marketing and advertising. To gauge the effectiveness of doctor branding efforts, it is essential to track and analyze the impact. It is recommended that every 2 to 3 years an introspective evaluation of the brand, the practice's positioning, its competitors, and the current local medical market be carried out to see if it may be time for a brand update or overhaul. Doctors can monitor online reviews, website traffic, social media engagement, and patient referrals. These data provide valuable insights into the success of branding strategies and helps identify areas for improvement.

The personal branding process takes work, and it is important that it is authentic. You can make your brand authentic and relatable by sharing personal values and writing in a way that allows your compassion and personality to shine through. Storytelling is often the key and can be used to a profound effect when sharing patient success stories, behind-the-scenes glimpses, or *day in the life* content.

This effort will help you better control your professional and personal image and the success and impact you can have as a leader. By following these steps, you can not only enhance your visibility and credibility but also unlock your unique abilities and potential.

## SUMMARY

Branding is a powerful method for dermatologists seeking professional success in their practice and providing leadership in their communities. By learning the methods of marketing and branding, physicians can provide an authentic and trusted voice to their patients and the public. Newer social media platforms can have a world-wide reach and require thoughtful and strategic use to persuade the public of the dermatologist's abilities, expertise, and leadership.

## CLINICS CARE POINTS

- Communication methods focused on authenticity and dedicated to patient care will improve patient satisfaction and increase public recognition because it builds trust.
- Branding can help deliver clear consistent messaging to patients and the public.
- Branding not only associates you with high-quality health care but can differentiate you from other practitioners.

## DISCLOSURE

The authors have no disclosure.

## REFERENCES

1. Branzetti J, Gisondi MA, Hopson LR, et al. Physician, know thyself: applying brand management principles to professional identity in academic medicine. Med Educ 2025;59(7):694–703.
2. "Your brand is what other people say about you when you're not in the room": what Jeff Bezos teaches professionals about reputation". The Times of India 2026.
3. Avery J, Greenwald R. A new approach to building your personal brand. Harv Bus Rev 2023. Available at: https://hbr.org/2023/05/a-new-approach-to-building-your-personal-brand. Accessed December 23, 2025.
4. Shryock T. What physicians need to know about marketing: what a strong personal brand looks like. Medicaleconomics.com. Medical Economics 2025. Available at: https://www.medicaleconomics.com/view/what-physicians-need-to-know-about-marketing-what-a-strong-personal-brand-looks-like. Accessed December 23, 2025.
5. Cronin TA, Cronin DW. Nice Guys and Girls Finish... First! 3 Boys Productions, ISBN 979-8-89480-721-8; 2024.
6. O'Reilly KB. 4 keys to marketing—and branding—your physician private practice. American Medical Association. 2023. Available at: https://www.ama-assn.org/practice-management/private-practices/4-keys-marketing-and-branding-your-physician-private-practice. Accessed December 23, 2025.
7. Building your doctor brand: Strategies for success. 2024. Sermo. Available at: https://www.sermo.com/resources/building-your-doctor-brand-strategies-for-success/. Accessed December 23, 2025.
8. Nyamathullah S. 12 doctor branding tips to succeed in medical practice. Hospital Success 2023. Available at: https://hospitalsuccess.com/12-doctor-branding-tips-to-succeed/. Accessed December 23, 2025.
9. Evans WD, Blitstein J, Vallone D, et al. Systematic review of health branding: growth of a promising practice. Transl Behav Med 2015;5(1):24–36.
10. MacArthur HV. The power of storytelling: inspiring and connecting with your audience. Forbes 2024. Available at: https://www.forbes.com/sites/hvmacarthur/2024/05/24/the-power-of-storytelling-inspiring-and-connecting-with-your-audience/. Accessed December 23, 2025.
11. Knott J. Branding for A medical practice & it's importance. Intrepy healthcare marketing. 2025. Available at: https://intrepy.com/branding-medical-practice-importance/. Accessed December 23, 2025.

12. Holinex Digital. The significance of personal brand promotion and management online. Linkedin.com 2023. Available at: https://www.linkedin.com/pulse/significance-personal-brand-promotion-management-online?utm_source=share&utm_medium=member_ios&utm_campaign=share_via. Accessed December 23, 2025.
13. Faria I, Cannada LK. Beyond the OR: building your niche and brand as a path to career growth in academic surgery. Am J Surg 2025116652. https://doi.org/10.1016/j.amjsurg.2025.116652.
14. Salokhe S. Branding healthcare: exploring effective approaches. Int J Healthc Manag 2025;1–11.
15. Pierre C. *Revenue boomers*. Revenue boomers. 2024. Available at: https://revenueboomers.com/blog/personal-branding-for-doctors/. Accessed December 23, 2025.
16. Morris O. *Physician branding*. Verify barrington. 2024. Available at: https://www.veritybarrington.com/physicianbranding. Accessed December 23, 2025.

# Creating a Culture of Inspiring Medical Leadership

Sabine Obagi, MD[a,*], Esther Wojcicki, PhD (hc)[b],
Arianne Shadi Kourosh, MD, MPH[c], Clay J. Cockerell, MD, MBA, JD[d]

**KEYWORDS**

• Medical leadership • Psychological safety • Mentorship • Team culture • Burnout
• Inclusive excellence • TRICK • Dermatology education

**KEY POINTS**

- Medical leadership operates on 2 levels: the microscopic, the physician shaping daily team culture, and the macroscopic, the specialty's shared responsibility for a thriving field.
- Freedom, dignity, and wealth - principles attributed to Cyrus the Great over 2500 years ago - offer a practical framework: give autonomy, defend dignity, and reward hard work.
- The TRICK framework (Trust, Respect, Independence, Collaboration, Kindness), developed by educator Esther Wojcicki, is readily exportable to medicine in treating patients, trainees, and team members.
- Advocating for a marginalized patient or defending a disrespected team member is among the highest-leverage actions a physician-leader can take, building lasting loyalty.
- The best physician-leaders do not need acknowledgment for the cultures they build; the highest compliment a team can give is: we did this ourselves.

## INTRODUCTION

> *Freedom, dignity, and wealth: give your people these three things and their love for you will never die.*
>
> —*Cyrus the Great*

There is a difference between a competent leader and an inspiring one. A competent leader manages effectively. An inspiring leader makes others want to be better, work harder, believe in a mission that extends beyond themselves. They make people feel that their work matters, and that they matter.

This article proposes that medical leadership operates on 2 distinct but inseparable levels. The first is microscopic: the attending physician whose daily decisions—how they enter a room, how they respond to a mistake, whether they defend a nurse being disrespected—set the tone for everyone watching. The second is macroscopic: leadership within a specialty.

How do we build community, on a medical team and in our specialty? How do we advocate for dermatology in ways that serve both physicians and patients? How do we create a culture of cohesion across institutions and training programs, one

Dedicated in memory of Susan Wojcicki (1968–2024), daughter of Esther Wojcicki, former CEO of YouTube, and inspiring leader.

[a] Department of Internal Medicine, Harbor-UCLA Medical Center, David Geffen School of Medicine at UCLA, 1000 West Carson Street, Torrance, CA 90502, USA; [b] Palo Alto, CA, USA; [c] Department of Dermatology, Harvard Medical School, Harvard TH Chan School of Public Health, Beth Israel Deaconess Medical Center, 330 Brookline Avenue, Boston, MA 02215, USA; [d] Cockerell Dermatopathology, HES/Lake Granbury Dermatology Residency, Department of Dermatology and Dermatopathology, UT Southwestern Medical Center, 2110 Research Row, Suite 100, Dallas, TX 75235, USA
* Corresponding author.
*E-mail address:* sabineobagi2026@gmail.com

Dermatol Clin 44 (2026) 633–640
https://doi.org/10.1016/j.det.2026.06.005


derm.theclinics.com

| Abbreviation | |
|---|---|
| TRICK | Trust, Respect, Independence, Collaboration, and Kindness |

that attracts and retains remarkable people rather than watching them leave for environments that make them feel seen?

Both levels are built from the same principles: trust, dignity, recognition, and the willingness to speak uncomfortable truths. This article is shaped by 4 vantage points: bedside medicine, academic dermatology, dermatopathology, and education, each clarifying what culture requires when the stakes are real.

## HISTORICAL PERSPECTIVES ON MEDICAL LEADERSHIP

The principles underlying inspiring medical leadership appear in consistent form across centuries and cultures, a powerful pattern worth noting.

### *Cyrus the Great and the Language of Human Dignity*

More than 2500 years ago, Cyrus the Great of Persia established what many historians consider the first charter of human rights.[1] What made his leadership endure was not military conquest but the culture he created: religious freedom, basic human dignity, and a direct sense of responsibility for the welfare of those under his authority.

> *Whenever you can, act as a liberator. Freedom, dignity, wealth—these three together constitute the greatest happiness of humanity. If you bequeath all three to your people, their love for you will never die.*[2]
>
> —*Cyrus the Great*

Freedom means autonomy: being trusted to contribute, to question, to lead. Dignity means modeling respect and being willing to defend it when others do not. Wealth, in the medical context, is not only monetary, but the experience that the leader of the team provides for the people under their care, provides for the needs and well-being of the people under the team and that their work leads to something, that their contribution is seen and valued. Wealth, in the medical field, involves making sure that people are provided for.

### *Hippocrates and the Guild of Medicine*

The Hippocratic Oath is widely known for its principle of nonmaleficence. Less appreciated is that this phrase does not actually appear in the original text; it was drawn from other Hippocratic writings and incorporated into later versions.[3] The original oath is about something else entirely:

> *To look upon his offspring in the same footing as my own brothers, and to teach them this art, if they shall wish to learn it, without fee or stipulation.*[4]
>
> —*Hippocrates*

Medicine is a guild, an order, a community of obligation. Those who have been given knowledge are bound to pass it on. Our actions—how we train the residents who will become tomorrow's attendings, how we treat the students watching us in clinic—affect everyone else in that order, whether we acknowledge it or not.

### *Dr Rudolf Virchow, Dr Paul Farmer, Dr Ernesto Gonzalez-Martinez, and the Tradition of Showing Up*

In the 19th century, Dr Rudolf Virchow was sent to investigate disease outbreaks in Silesia. His findings were politically explosive when he concluded that the epidemic was spreading because of poverty, overcrowding, and a government's failure to care for its people.[5] "Physicians are the natural attorneys of the poor," he wrote. He became a model for Dr Paul Farmer, who would build Partners in Health on the same conviction.[6] Dr Farmer did not build Partners in Health, an international nonprofit public health organization, by being the most talented physician in the room. He built it by creating a culture so clear in its purpose that people chose to work in the hardest conditions on Earth because they believed in what they were building together. *Mountains Beyond Mountains*, Tracy Kidder's biography, takes its name from a Haitian proverb that one author of this article encouraged another to read: "beyond every mountain, there is another."[6] The work is never finished. What matters is whether you have built a culture in which others can keep climbing after you.

In dermatology, this concept was embodied by Dr Ernesto Gonzalez-Martinez, the first Hispanic dermatologist at Massachusetts General Hospital and Harvard Medical School. Raised with limited resources in Puerto Rico, he understood the weight of social determinants of health. He established a free dermatology clinic through the Boston Health Care for the Homeless Program, pioneered free telemedicine for underserved populations in Puerto Rico and Honduras, and founded the first mentorship program for underrepresented minority medical students in the country.[7] He described his life's work not as sacrifice, but as "service as an avocation." When he retired, those who trained under him committed to carrying his legacy forward, which is, perhaps, the most honest measure of a culture well built.

## *Esther Wojcicki and the Origins of the TRICK Method*

Esther Wojcicki, PhD—an educator, journalist, and co-author of this article—spent nearly four decades teaching at Palo Alto High School. She has been affectionately called the "Godmother of Silicon Valley," a title that is the subject of a recent documentary with the same name, and appropriately earned through building: a journalism program, a philosophy of trust, a generation of students who went on to reshape the world,[8,9] 2 of whom are her daughter Susan Wojcicki, former CEO of YouTube, and Anne Wojcicki, co-founder and CEO of 23andMe—women whose careers reflect what their mother had been practicing in a classroom for decades.

This matters for medicine because what Dr Wojcicki created was a culture of intellectual freedom and psychological safety. When people feel trusted and respected, they feel free enough to take intellectual and emotional risks: they speak up, admit mistakes, and ask questions.[10] On a medical team, residents, nurses, and staff who fear judgment may withhold concerns. In the best case, that silence limits innovation and perspective. In the worst case, it masks errors that become adverse events. Research demonstrates that teams lacking psychological safety show diminished learning behaviors and impaired ability to implement new practices safely.[11–13]

What Dr Wojcicki built defies most assumptions about what is supposed to happen in a classroom. Her journalism program grew at a pace that alarmed the school administration. Students who had no reason to stay late were arriving early, year after year. The administration, unable to explain it, accused her of giving students pizza as an incentive. She found the accusation amusing, as she was not bribing anyone, but rather creating a space where people felt cared for and wanted to be.

When Dr Wojcicki finally asked her students why they kept coming back, what they said surprised her. "You trust us," they told her. She assumed this was universal. "Doesn't everybody trust you?" she asked. They told her they felt no one else in the school trusted or respected them, that they felt like they were being watched constantly, and treated as potential problems to contain instead of as people capable of remarkable things. In 40 years of teaching, Esther never sent a single student to the principal's office for misbehavior. Not a single one.

This is where the TRICK method solidified. Trust, Respect, Independence, Collaboration, and Kindness are the key elements developed by a teacher who reflected on what she was doing and asked her students to help put it into words.[8] TRICK is a description of what high-performing cultures already do intuitively from the inside. Dr Wojcicki gave that state of being a name.

The reach of the TRICK framework was profound. Her students' newspaper won first place in the nation year after year and has since grown to 14 publications. Larry Page and Sergey Brin founded Google in the garage of Dr Wojcicki's daughter Susan, and the culture of that company bears the unmistakable imprint of what Esther had been building a few miles away.[8] Susan Wojcicki moved from Intel, where employees clocked in and out and sensors tracked time spent in chairs, to Google, where offices were glass, hours were flexible, meals were prepared on site, and 20% of work time was given freely to self-directed projects. Two of those 20-percent projects became Gmail and Google Maps. The contrast between Intel and Google was apparent. Every structural decision at Google communicated the same message of trust. The culture of trust and safety creates intellectual risk and honesty necessary for real innovation.

Dr Wojcicki learned this from a tragedy. As a child, she watched her mother, an immigrant woman who had been taught to defer to authority, follow a physician's instructions after her youngest brother, as a toddler, ingested a bottle of aspirin. The physician, not listening carefully, told her to put him to bed and wait. She was afraid to ask another question. The authority of the physician felt absolute. By the time 2 hours had passed, he was violently ill. He did not survive. Esther has spent her life teaching students, and later her own children, to ask the difficult question no matter what, because people in authority do not always have the right answer, even when they speak as though they do.

In a medical context, this is a patient safety imperative. Patients who feel unable to question their physicians, and staff who feel unable to question their attendings, create conditions of preventable harm.

Dr Wojcicki's daughter Susan Wojcicki understood this from the inside. At Google, she built and led Google Video before going to the board and telling them directly that she had spent a billion dollars on a product that was not working, and that she now wanted to spend $1.3 billion to acquire YouTube instead. "Most leaders would not do that," recalled Esther. The same culture that taught her to speak up as a child was reinforced at a school board meeting where her mother was challenging the English department. It was the culture that gave her the standing to say the uncomfortable thing in a boardroom decades later. Shortly before her death in 2024, Susan wrote that the greatest gift her mother gave her was the ability to think independently and not always defer to experts. "When you speak out," she wrote, "people take you more seriously. That is a good thing."[14] It is a sentence that belongs in every medical school orientation.

## Lao Tzu and the Tao Te Ching

The Tao Te Ching has influenced leaders and physicians for more than 2000 years. Dr Clay Cockerell has drawn on it throughout his career, presenting its lessons for dermatology at the American Academy of Dermatology and the Dallas Dermatologic Society.[15]

> *A leader is best when people barely know that he exists. But of a good leader, who talks little, when his work is done, his aim fulfilled, they will all say: we did this ourselves.*[16]
>
> —*Lao Tzu, Tao Te Ching, Verse 17 (translated by Witter Bynner).*

These verses point to the same truth as Cyrus and Hippocrates: the leader who serves, who does not grasp for credit, who makes space for others to grow, builds something that outlasts any individual career.

### Freedom as autonomy, trust, and the culture of voice

The first element of inspiring leadership culture is freedom: the experience, by every member of a team, of being trusted to contribute, to question, and to lead within their role. Research in organizational psychology consistently shows that team performance is less predicted by the average ability of its members than by the quality of their shared culture.[10] The most reliably high-performing teams share what researchers call psychological safety, the shared belief that the team is safe for interpersonal risk-taking.[10]

The stakes in medicine are high. From the scrub technician who notices a count discrepancy but stays silent because the attending has never welcomed interruption, to the first-year resident who sees a wrong site on a surgical consent but does not speak up because they have learned what happens when they do, these silences are a failure of freedom, and each is a moment when team culture became a patient safety risk.[13]

Dr Wojcicki's story about the loss of her brother makes painfully clear that this dynamic extends to patients as well. "That imprinted me for life," Wojcicki said. "I teach people to ask the difficult questions no matter what the circumstance is."

Almost weekly, those of us in medicine may encounter patients who feel intimidated by the white coat, patients who have been made to feel that their questions are an imposition. Dr Kourosh has described patients thanking her for never expressing frustration when they arrive with Internet printouts and long lists of questions. Her response is always the same: patients who ask questions tend to do better. They get well.

Freedom is built through small behaviors, such as asking the medical student what they think before giving the answer, or saying openly, "I may be wrong here, does anyone see this differently?" Freedom in leadership means empowering people to lead within their role, such as the attending who gives a resident genuine ownership of a project, or a program director who asks junior faculty to chair a committee. Each of these builds the kind of loyalty no salary structure can replicate.

### Dignity as respect, protection, and the courage to defend

Dignity operates on 2 levels: modeling, and protection. Modeling, which can be expressed as an attending who greets every team member by name, who listens as carefully to the medical student as to the fellow, who does not dismiss the nurse's observation, is teaching through every interaction. The residents watching will carry it forward.

The second part of dignity is protection. The inspiring leader defends the dignity of their team when others do not, requiring a courage rarely discussed in leadership training: the willingness to have uncomfortable conversations. A patient may sometimes speak to nurses and staff in ways that are demeaning, or vice versa. The attending who witnesses it and says nothing teaches everyone in the room that dignity is conditional. The attending who steps in, calmly and directly, teaches something entirely different.

> *The loyalty that team members feel when they see that you actually stood up for them is unparalleled. It is the kind of loyalty that no salary adjustment can produce.*
>
> —*Dr Arianne Shadi Kourosh*

Dignity also shapes how we respond to a patient who may question our recommendations. The pediatrician who cared for Dr Wojcicki's family told her: there is nobody who knows their child better than the mother. When another doctor told Dr Wojcicki to give her daughter a preventive antibiotic before an infection had even developed, she resisted. Her daughter recovered without it. Years later, prophylactic antibiotics for mildly red ears would cease to be standard practice altogether.[17] The mother who asked the question was right. The culture that made it safe to ask was the work of one physician who respected her judgment enough to say so.

### *Recognition as the modern form of wealth*

> *I didn't have control over how much the nurses were paid. But I could make sure they were recognized.*
>
> *—Dr Arianne Shadi Kourosh*

Wealth, as a leadership principle, is the principle that hard work leads to something, that effort is seen, contribution is recognized, and the people who provide extraordinary care will not go unnoticed. The failure to recognize effort is one of the clearest drivers of burnout and disengagement across medicine.[18]

Dr Kourosh describes nominating nurses and staff for institutional awards, a practice that many busy physicians may not take time to do.[18] One nurse, upon winning a hospital-wide award, told her that the recognition meant more than any raise she had ever received, because what the nomination said was: your work was seen.

Dr Wojcicki's classroom ran the same way. Every 2 weeks, when a new edition of the student newspaper came out, the class held a structured public critique. She had students lead it. They named what had worked before naming what could improve. Nobody was embarrassed, Esther said, because the culture made it clear that one is capable, one just needs to know how and to be given the opportunity. The publications won first place nationally, year after year. That consistency was produced by a culture that attributed success openly and treated everyone in the room as someone capable of outstanding work, rather than by talent alone.

Data presented at the 2026 American Academy of Dermatology Annual Meeting showed that dermatologists now receive an average of 49 patient portal messages per day, up more than 50% since 2020, the vast majority uncompensated.[19] Women physicians receive 26% more of these messages and spend 20% more time in the inbox. The connection to burnout is direct. Physician-leaders who understand wealth as a cultural value work to correct it at every level available to them, and they also invest in pipeline programs, nominate junior colleagues for awards and committee positions, and expand the circle of who gets to belong to the profession.[20–22]

## THE DERMATOLOGIST AS A CULTURE LEADER

### *In the Clinic*

The clinic is where culture originates. An attending who pauses after a complex case to debrief with the resident, who greets the front desk staff with the same warmth extended to patients, who creates space for clinical uncertainty to be named rather than masked, is building a collaborative leadership culture. The decisions made when no one appears to be watching are, in fact, watched by everyone.

### *In Dermatopathology Sign-out*

Dermatopathology sign-out represents one of the richest opportunities for culture-building in all of dermatology. Dr Clay Cockerell, who has personally diagnosed more than 3 million biopsies and trained generations of dermatopathologists, described the philosophy at the heart of this work: that one cannot read a slide without understanding the person it came from. The argument for clinicopathologic correlation is, at its root, an argument about connection over isolation. The dermatopathologist who may call the submitting clinician because the patient's story is inseparable from the slide is modeling what it looks like to refuse the convenience of working in silos to every trainee in the room. He who creates space for the junior resident's interpretation, taking it seriously, and naming what was before offering a correction, models the intellectual generosity that, quietly, and repeated over thousands of cases, is building inspiring cultural leadership.

### *In Dermatology and the HIV Epidemic*

The human immunodeficiency virus (HIV) epidemic in the 1980s was a moment that asked dermatology, and dermatopathology specifically, to show up for something frightening and stigmatized before the clinical picture was even fully understood. Cutaneous manifestations were often among the earliest findings in acquired immunodeficiency syndrome (AIDS)-related illness, meaning that biopsies and their interpretation were central to care.[23] Dr Cockerell's philosophy—that you cannot read a slide without understanding the person it came from—was precisely the orientation that moment demanded. The willingness to stay connected to the whole patient, rather than retreat into the slide alone, was—in addition to being a clinical necessity, a cultural act not unlike what Dr Virchow did in Silesia or Dr Farmer in Haiti displayed in showing up for the hardest problem when others may have looked away.

### In Academic Medicine and Professional Organizations

Academic dermatologists shape the culture of the specialty through the trainees they educate and the norms they embody. Faculty who assign authorship fairly, teach research methodology explicitly, and connect trainees to their professional networks accelerate leadership development.[24] This is how culture compounds.

Professional societies are also powerful. Their leadership structures, award cultures, and programming priorities send clear signals about what the field values. Dermatologists engaging with these organizations shape the culture of the field, advocate for representation, sponsor emerging leaders, and embody macroscopic leadership.

## WHAT SELFLESS LEADERSHIP ACTUALLY LOOKS LIKE

When asked what defined a great leader, Dr Cockerell answered without hesitation: servant leadership. In a career spanning nearly 4 decades, encompassing more than 3 million biopsies diagnosed, a residency program founded, 4 graduate degrees earned, and the presidency of the American Academy of Dermatology, the answer was simple: the leader exists to serve the people around them, not the other way around.

> *Without taking credit, is accredited. Laying no claim, is acclaimed. And because he does not compete, finds peaceful competence.*[15,16]
>
> *—Lao Tzu, Tao Te Ching, Verse 22 (translated by Witter Bynner).*

This is the philosophy of what the best physician-leaders actually look like when you work alongside them. They do not need acknowledgment for the cultures they build, but are simply building them, one interaction at a time, because that is what the work demands.

Dr Wojcicki described the same orientation from the perspective of education. The leaders she has watched succeed are the ones who created environments where everyone else could do their best work and then stepped back. When people feel trusted, she said, they work harder for you than any management system can compel. When they feel respected as whole persons, they bring dimensions of themselves to their work that never would have appeared under surveillance.

Burnout affects an estimated 40% to 60% of practicing physicians.[18] Leaders who are burned out cannot model energy, generosity, or purpose. Addressing burnout is an investment in the capacity to lead.

## PRACTICAL TOOLS FOR BUILDING INSPIRING LEADERSHIP CULTURE

Culture is what happens in the 10 seconds after someone speaks up. In those seconds, leaders teach people whether voice is safe. Inspiring culture is built through small behaviors, consistently practiced.

Explicit invitations for inclusion. In every meeting or case discussion, invite the quietest voice: I would love to hear your read on this. Over time, this normalizes broad participation.

Public attribution. When a team member's observation contributes to a good outcome, name it.

Attribution is one of the lowest-cost, highest-impact currencies of leadership.

Nominating colleagues for awards. Institutional awards exist at every hospital and academic center. Some physicians may not take the time. The ones who do create a culture where effort is visibly valued.

Structured critique and reflection. A public, student-led critique after every publication, as Dr Wojcicki ran for 40 years, is a model worth borrowing: name what worked before naming what could improve. Adapted to case conferences or postprocedure debriefs, it builds learning cultures over time.

Defending dignity in the room. When a patient or visitor treats a team member with disrespect, address it directly and respectfully. The loyalty this builds is unlike anything a compensation structure can produce.

Structured individual check-ins. Brief, regular conversations with team members—focused beyond task status to include well-being and development—build the relational trust that psychological safety requires.

## SUMMARY

The most inspiring leaders in dermatology are the ones who understood that their greatest contribution is not what they built for themselves, but what they make possible for others. From Cyrus the Great to Dr Paul Farmer, from the Hippocratic guild to the cultures that produced Gmail and YouTube, the message is consistent: freedom, dignity, and wealth, given to the people who work alongside us every day, produce something that neither talent nor technology can manufacture. They produce the kind of loyalty, creativity, and courage that defines a team worth belonging to.[6,8,10,11]

The question for each of us—in every clinic, every sign-out room, every department meeting—is the same question Dr Farmer and Dr Virchow and Cyrus the Great were answering in their own time: what kind of culture am I building? And what will I do today, in the small decisions that no one may notice, to build it?

## CLINICS CARE POINTS

- Medical leadership operates on 2 levels: the microscopic (the attending physician as daily architect of team culture) and the macroscopic (the specialty's collective responsibility to build a field where physicians and patients thrive). Both require intentional, consistent effort.
- Psychological safety—the shared belief that the team environment is safe for interpersonal risk-taking—is one of the most predictive factors of high-performing medical teams and a direct patient safety imperative.[10,11,13] It is built through small, consistent behaviors.
- Freedom, dignity, and wealth—giving your people autonomy, defending their dignity, and ensuring their hard work is recognized—are the practical foundation of inspiring leadership culture, applicable in any practice setting regardless of resources. The original Hippocratic tradition embodies mentorship and guild: medicine as an order, the obligation to the people we train, and to the colleagues who trained us.
- Public attribution, nominating colleagues for awards, and defending team members in difficult moments cost nothing and build the kind of loyalty that no compensation structure can produce.
- The results of both the philosophy of Cyrus the Great and the TRICK method are the same: creating a culture of safety and feeling cared for, and therefore performing with the highest level of intellectual honesty. And carrying forward the inspiring mission of medicine.

## DISCLOSURE

The authors report no commercial or financial conflicts of interest and no funding sources to disclose.

## REFERENCES

1. United Nations. Replica of the "Edict of Cyrus." UN gifts, MIT Classics Hippocratic Oath translation. Available at: https://www.un.org/ungifts/replica-edict-cyrus. Accessed May 16, 2026.
2. Xenophenon. Xenophon's Cyrus the Great: The Arts of Leadership and War [book]. Hedrick L, editor. New York, NY: Truman Talley Books/St. Martin's Press; 2006:116. Also cited in: Plutarch. The Age of Alexander [book]. Scott-Kilvert I, translator. London: Penguin; 1973:326.
3. Smith S. Origin and uses of primum non nocere — above all, do no harm! J Clin Pharmacol 2005;45(4): 371–7.
4. Hippocrates. The oath. Translated by Adams F. ca. 400 BCE. Available at: https://classics.mit.edu/Hippocrates/hippooath.html. Accessed May 16, 2026.
5. Virchow RC. Report on the typhus epidemic in upper silesia. Am J Publ Health 2006;96(12):2102–5.
6. Kidder T. Mountains beyond Mountains: the quest of Dr. Paul Farmer, a man who would cure the world. New York: Random House; 2003.
7. Santiago Mangual KP, Patin EA, Kourosh AS. Dermatologists carrying forward the legacy of Rudolf Virchow: lessons learned from Dr. Ernesto Gonzalez-Martinez. J Am Acad Dermatol 2025;92(5): 1176–8.
8. Wojcicki E. How to raise successful people: simple lessons for radical results. Boston: Houghton Mifflin Harcourt; 2019.
9. The Godmother of Silicon Valley: The Teacher Who Changed the World [documentary film]. 2026.
10. Edmondson A. Psychological safety and learning behavior in work teams. Adm Sci Q 1999;44(2): 350–83.
11. Edmondson AC, Bohmer RM, Pisano GP. Disrupted routines: team learning and new technology implementation in hospitals. Adm Sci Q 2001;46(4): 685–716.
12. Edmondson AC. The fearless organization: creating psychological safety in the workplace for learning, innovation, and growth. Hoboken (NJ): Wiley; 2018.
13. Leape LL, Berwick DM. Five years after to err is human: what have we learned? JAMA 2005;293(19): 2384–90.
14. Wojcicki S. What I learned from my mom. In: Dunn JD, Westin SR, editors. What I learned from mom. New York: Simon & Schuster; 2025.
15. Cockerell CJ. Pressure and disenchantment in physicians-part II: lessons for physicians from the Tao Te Ching. Clin Dermatol 2017;35(1):100–4.
16. Laozi. The way of life according to Lao-tzu. Translated by Bynner W. New York: Perigee Books; 1944.
17. Lieberthal AS, Carroll AE, Chonmaitree T, et al. The diagnosis and management of acute otitis media. Pediatrics 2013;131(3):e964–99.
18. Shanafelt TD, West CP, Sinsky C, et al. Changes in burnout and satisfaction with work-life integration in physicians and the general US working population between 2011 and 2020. Mayo Clin Proc 2022; 97(3):491–506.

19. Gracey Maniar LE. Surge in unbilled patient-initiated portal messages: implications for physician compensation and burnout. Presented at: American Academy of Dermatology Annual Meeting; 2026; Denver, CO. Cited in: Grasso A. Healio. April 8, 2026.
20. Cline A, Winter RP, Kourosh S, et al. Multiethnic training in residency: a survey of dermatology residents. Cutis 2020;105(6):310–3.
21. Pollock S, Taylor S, Kourosh AS, et al. The dark side of skin lightning: an international collaboration and review of a public health issue affecting dermatology. Int J Womens Dermatol 2021;7(2):158–64.
22. Santiago Mangual KP, Gochnauer H, Kourosh AS. Color me unhealthy: the toxic health effects of colorism. J Am Acad Dermatol 2024;91(6):1299–300.
23. Cockerell CJ. The changing spectrum of the cutaneous manifestations of HIV disease. Arch Dermatol 1998;134(11):1385–6.
24. Patton EW, Griffith KA, Jones RD, et al. Differences in mentor-mentee sponsorship in male vs female recipients of National Institutes of Health grants. JAMA Intern Med 2017;177(4):580–2.

United States Postal Service

# Statement of Ownership, Management and Circulation
## (All Periodicals Publications Except Requester Publications)

| 1. Publication Title | 2. Publication Number | 3. Filing Date |
|---|---|---|
| DERMATOLOGIC CLINICS | 0 0 0 - 7 0 5 | 08/24/2026 |
| **4. Issue Frequency** | **5. Number of Issues Published Annually** | **6. Annual Subscription Price** |
| JAN, APR, JUL, OCT | 4 | $456.00 |

7. Complete Mailing Address of Known Office of Publication (Not printer) (Street, city, county, state, and ZIP+4)
Addr 1: Elsevier INC
Addr 2: 230 Park Ave Ste 800
City, State ZIP: New York NY 10169

Contact Person: Mohana Priya Damodharan
Telephone: 91-44-4299-4077

8. Complete Mailing Address of Headquarters or General Business Office of Publisher (Not Printer)
Addr 1: Elsevier INC
Addr 2: 230 Park Ave Ste 800
City, State ZIP: New York NY 10169

9. Full Names and Complete Mailing Addresses of Publisher, Editor and Managing Editor (do not leave blank)

Publisher (Name and complete mailing address)
Name: Dolores Meloni, ELSEVIER INC.
Addr 1: 1600 JOHN F KENNEDY BLVD. SUITE 1600
Addr 2:
City, State ZIP: PHILADELPHIA, PA 19103-2899

Editor (Name and complete mailing address)
Name: STACY EASTMAN, ELSEVIER INC.
Addr 1: 1600 JOHN F KENNEDY BLVD. SUITE 1600
Addr 2:
City, State ZIP: PHILADELPHIA, PA 19103-2899

Managing Editor (Name and complete mailing address)
Name: PATRICK MANLEY, ELSEVIER INC.
Addr 1: 1600 JOHN F KENNEDY BLVD. SUITE 1600
Addr 2:
City, State ZIP: PHILADELPHIA, PA 19103-2899

10. Owner (Do not leave blank. If the publication is owned by a corporation, give the name and address of the corporation immediately followed by the names and addresses of all stockholders owning or holding 1 Percent or more of the total amount of stock. If not owned by a corporation, give the names and addresses of all the individual owners. If owned by a partnership or other unincorporated firm, give it's name and address as well as those of each individual owner. If the publication is published by a nonprofit organization, give it's name and address.)

| Full Name | Complete Mailing Address |
|---|---|
| WHOLLY OWNED SUBSIDIARY OF REED/ELSEVIER, | 1600 JOHN F KENNEDY BLVD. SUITE 1600 |
| US HOLDINGS | PHILADELPHIA, PA 19103-2899 |

11. Known Bondholders, Mortgagees and Other Security Holders Owning or Holding 1 Percent or more of Total Amount of Bonds, Mortgages, or Other Securities. If none, check box → ☐ None

| Full Name | Complete Mailing Address |
|---|---|
| NA | |

12. Tax Status (For completion by nonprofit organizations authorized to mail at nonprofit rates) (Check one)
The purpose, function, and nonprofit status of this organization and the exempt status for federal income tax purposes:
[X] Has Not changed During Preceding 12 Months
[ ] Has Changed During Preceding 12 Months (Publisher must submit explanation of change with this statement below)



| 13. Publication Title | | | 14. Issue Date for Circulation Data Below | |
|---|---|---|---|---|
| DERMATOLOGIC CLINICS | | | October 2026 | |
| 15. **Extent and Nature of Circulation** | | | **Average No. Copies Each Issue During Preceding 12 Months** | **No. Copies of Single Issue Published Nearest to filing Date** |
| a. Total Number of Copies (Net press run) | | | 93 | 79 |
| b. Paid and/or Requested Circulation | (1) | Mailed Outside-County Paid Subscriptions Stated on PS Form 3541 (Include paid distribution above nominal rate, advertiser's proof copies, and exchange copies) | 42 | 27 |
| | (2) | Mailed In-County Paid Subscriptions Stated on PS Form 3541 (Include paid distribution above nominal rate, advertiser's proof copies, and exchange copies) | 0 | 0 |
| | (3) | Paid Distribution Outside the Mails Including Sales Through Dealers and Carriers, Street Vendors, Counter Sales ,and Other Paid Distribution Ouside USPS | 34 | 33 |
| | (4) | Paid Distribution by Other Classes of Mail Through the USPS (e.g. First-Class Mail) | 10 | 12 |
| c. Total Paid Distribution [Sum of 15b. (1), (2), (3), and (4)] ▶ | | | 86 | 72 |
| d. Free or Nominal Rate Distribution (By Mail and Outside the Mail) | (1) | Free or Nominal Rate Outside-County Copies Included on PS Form 3541 | 6 | 6 |
| | (2) | Free or Nominal In-County Copies Included on PS Form 3541 | 0 | 0 |
| | (3) | Free or Nominal Rate Copies Mailed at Other Classes Through the USPS (e.g. First-Class Mail) | 0 | 0 |
| | (4) | Free or Nominal Rate Distribution Outside the Mail (Carriers or other means) | 1 | 1 |
| e. Total Free or Nominal Rate Distribution (Sum of 15d. (1), (2), (3) and (4)) ▶ | | | 7 | 7 |
| f. Total Distribution (Sum of 15c. and 15e.) ▶ | | | 93 | 79 |
| g. Copies not Distributed (See Instructions to Publishers #4 (page #3)) | | | 0 | 0 |
| h. Total (Sum of 15f. and g.) ▶ | | | 93 | 79 |
| i. Percent Paid (15c. Divided by 15f. Times 100) ▶ | | | 92.47% | 91.14% |

* if you are claiming electronic copies, go to line 16 on page 3. If you are not claiming electronic copies, skip to line 17 on page 3.

| 16. Electronic copy Circulation | | |
|---|---|---|
| If present, check box → | | |
| a. Paid Electronic Copies | | |
| b. Total Paid Print Copies (Line 15c) + Paid Electronic Copies (Line 16a) ▶ | 86 | 72 |
| c. Total Print Distribution (Line 15F) + Paid Electronic Copies (Line 16a) ▶ | 93 | 79 |
| d. Percentage Paid (Both Print & Electronic Copies (16b divided bt 16c x 100) ▶ | 92.47% | 91.14% |

[X] I certify that 50% of all my distribution copies (electronic and Print) are paid above a nominal price

17. Publication of Statement of Ownership
[X] Publication required. Will be printed in the **October 2026** issue of this publication. [ ] Publication not required

| 18. Signature and Title of Editor, Publisher, Business Manager, or Owner | Title | Date |
|---|---|---|
| Mohana Priya Damodharan | Distribution Controller | 8/24/2026 |

I certify that all information furnished on this form is true and complete. I understand that anyone who furnishes false or misleading information on this form or who omits material or information requested on the form may be subject to criminal sanctions (including fines and imprisonment) and/or civil sanctions (including civil penalties)

9780443429651